D1756772

FRCS General Su
Section 1

500 SBAs and EMIs

SECOND EDITION

FRCS General Surgery Section 1

500 SBAs and EMIs

SECOND EDITION

Alasdair Wilson MBChB MSc MD FRCSEd
Consultant in Vascular Surgery
Aberdeen Royal Infirmary
Clinical Lecturer in General Surgery
University of Aberdeen, UK

Diane Hildebrand BSc MBChB FRCS
Specialty Registrar in General Surgery
Aberdeen Royal Infirmary
University of Aberdeen, UK

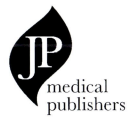

JP
medical
publishers

London • Panama City • New Delhi

ISBN: 978-1-909836-69-3

British Library Cataloguing in Publication Data
A catalogue record for this book is available from the British Library

Library of Congress Cataloging in Publication Data
A catalog record for this book is available from the Library of Congress

Commissioning Editor: Steffan Clements
Editorial Assistant: Adam Rajah
Design: Designers Collective Ltd

Foreword

I have known the authors of the second edition of *FRCS General Surgery Section 1: 500 SBAs and EMIs* for more than a decade and both of them have a strong commitment to teaching, education and training. They have developed this book based on their own experience of taking the FRCS exam and in their current role as trainers, mentoring senior trainees preparing for the fellowship exam.

The second edition of *FRCS General Surgery Section 1: 500 SBAs and EMIs* provides practice questions that mirror the style used in the FRCS General Surgery: Section 1, which is a written examination with both single best answer and extended matching item question formats. The questions have been developed carefully to test the reader's knowledge base, and more importantly to assess their reasoning ability and judgment. These are key skills for passing the exam.

The range of topics covered in the questions also provides useful guidance for building an essential knowledge base. The book is divided into chapters reflecting the subspecialties in general surgery so that candidates preparing for the exam can consolidate their knowledge in an organised manner. The first edition of the book addressed the sparse availability of practice questions for the FRCS examination. The second edition has been updated to reflect the changes in best surgical practice and the current examination syllabus.

Passing the FRCS exam requires many skills, but inevitably involves practice and familiarity with the style and format of the examination. This book undoubtedly provides a valuable adjunct for candidates during this process.

Emad H Aly MBBCh MD FRCS FACS FASCRS MEd FFSTEd
Consultant Colorectal and General Surgeon
Aberdeen Royal Infirmary
Aberdeen, UK
Honorary Clinical Senior Lecturer
University of Aberdeen
Aberdeen, UK

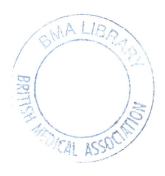

Preface

The FRCS General Surgery Section 1 examination consists of two papers, and a combined pass from both is required to proceed to Section 2. Paper 1 consists of multiple choice questions and lasts two hours. Paper 2 consists of extended matching item questions and lasts two and a half hours. The questions are predominantly scenario-based and are designed to cover the breadth of the current Intercollegiate Surgical Curriculum.

FRCS General Surgery Section 1: 500 SBAs and EMIs provides practice questions for the candidate sitting the Section 1 examination. The book offers up-to-date, comprehensive coverage of the entire curriculum and the questions are written in the same style as those in the exam. It is structured according to surgical specialties (general and emergency, breast, colorectal, endocrine, hepatobiliary, transplantation, upper gastrointestinal, and vascular and endovascular) and incorporates the two question formats from both papers.

For the second edition, we have replaced fifty questions and revised many others to bring the book up to date with the curriculum, and to reflect changes in modern surgical practice.

Because candidates have two years from their first attempt to gain eligibility to proceed to Section 2 (with a maximum of four attempts), we believe time spent preparing with this revision aid is invaluable, not just to maximise the chances of passing first time, but also of passing well.

Good luck!

Alasdair Wilson
Diane Hildebrand
March 2018

Contents

Glossary

AAT	Alanine amino transaminase
ABPI	Ankle brachial pressure index
αFP	Alpha fetoprotein
ANOVA	Analysis of variance
APACHE II	Acute physiology & chronic health evaluation
ASA	American Society of Anesthesiologists
ATLS	Advanced trauma life support
β-hCG	Beta-human chorionic gonadotrophin
BMI	Body mass index
CBD	Common bile duct
CABG	Coronary artery bypass graft
CEA	Carcinoembryonic antigen
CEAP	Clinical/(a)etiologic/anatomical/pathophysiological
CPEX	Cardiopulmonary exercise testing
CRP	C-reactive protein
CT	Computed tomography
CTA	Computed tomography angiography
DSA	Digital subtraction angiography
ELISA	Enzyme-linked immunosorbent assay
ERCP	Endoscopic retrograde cholangiopancreatography
FDG-PET	Fluorodeoxyglucose positron emission tomography
GGT	Gamma glutamyl transaminase
HDU	High dependency unit
HLA	Human leukocyte antigen
ISS	Injury severity score
IVDA	Intravenous drug abuser
kPa	Kilopascals
LFT	Liver function test
METS	Metabolic equivalent task score
MODS	Multiple organ dysfunction syndrome
MRA	Magnetic resonance angiography
MRCP	Magnetic resonance cholangiopancreatography
MUGA	Multi-gated acquisition scan
O-POSSUM	Oesophagogastric physiological and operative score for the numeration of mortality and morbidity
P-POSSUM	Physiological and operative score for the numeration of mortality and morbidity
Pa_{O_2/CO_2}	Partial arterial pressure of oxygen/carbon dioxide
PFT	Pulmonary function test
PTA	Percutaneous transluminal angioplasty
PTC	Percutaneous transhepatic cholangiography

RTS	Revised trauma score
SAPS II	Simplified acute physiology score
SIRS	Systemic inflammatory response syndrome
TNM	Tumour–nodes–metastases
TOS	Thoracic outlet syndrome
UNOS	United Network for Organ Sharing
VACTERL	Vertebral anomalies, anal atresia, cardiovascular anomalies, tracheo-oesophageal fistula, renal abnormalities, limb defects

Recommended reading

Beard JD, Gaines PA and Loftus I (eds). Vascular and Endovascular Surgery: A Companion to Specialist Surgical Practice, 5th edition. Philadelphia: Saunders, Elsevier, 2014.

Dixon JM (ed). Breast Surgery: A Companion to Specialist Surgical Practice, 5th edition. Philadelphia: Saunders, Elsevier, 2014.

Forsyth JLR (ed). Transplantation: A Companion to Specialist Surgical Practice, 5th edition. Philadelphia: Saunders, Elsevier, 2014.

Garden OJ and Parks RW (ed). Hepatobiliary and Pancreatic Surgery: A Companion to Specialist Surgical Practice, 5th edition. Philadelphia: Saunders, Elsevier, 2014.

Griffin SM, Raimes SA and Shenfine J (eds). Oesophagogastric Surgery: A Companion to Specialist Surgical Practice, 5th edition. Philadelphia: Saunders, Elsevier, 2014.

Jones PF, Krukowski ZH and Youngson GG (eds). Emergency Abdominal Surgery, 3rd edition. London: Chapman and Hall Medical, 1998.

Lennard TWJ (ed). Endocrine Surgery: A Companion to Specialist Surgical Practice, 5th edition. Philadelphia: Saunders, Elsevier, 2014.

Paterson-Brown S (ed). Core Topics in General and Emergency Surgery: A Companion to Specialist Surgical Practice, 5th edition. Philadelphia: Saunders, Elsevier, 2014.

Philips RKS and Clark S (ed). Colorectal Surgery: A Companion to Specialist Surgical Practice, 5th edition. Philadelphia: Saunders, Elsevier, 2014.

Further details of the exam regulations can be found on the ISB website: www.intercollegiate.org. uk. We recommend reading the content of this website in advance of the exam, since it provides important information on registration for the day of the exam.

Acknowledgements

The production of this book would not have been possible without the extensive work done by the previous authors and editors, and the publisher. We would especially like to thank Ms. Lynn Stevenson and Miss Wendy Craig for their large contributions to the first edition. I would also like to thank my wife Fiona for her constant support and understanding.

AW

I extend my thanks to the previous authors, editors and the publisher for their work, as well as to Mr Alasdair Wilson for his continuing advice and encouragement, not only in the production of this volume, but throughout my career. I would also like to thank Bob for his endless encouragement and patience.

DH

Chapter 1

General and emergency surgery

Questions: SBAs

For each question, select the single best answer from the five options listed.

1. An 85-year-old woman presents with a 6-hour history of severe sudden onset central abdominal pain. Her heart rate is 110 beats per minute and irregular. Her blood pressure is 132/94 mmHg and temperature is 38.1°C. Abdominal examination reveals a generally soft but distended and tender abdomen with no audible bowel sounds. Per rectal examination reveals guaiac-positive stool.

   What is the most likely diagnosis?

   A   Abdominal aortic aneurysm
   B   Acute pancreatitis
   C   Mesenteric ischaemia
   D   Myocardial infarction
   E   Peptic ulcer disease

2. In patients who present with acute pancreatitis, which factor is least likely to independently predict the development of complications?

   A   Age > 55 years
   B   APACHE II score > 8 points in the first 24 hours of admission
   C   C-reactive protein > 150 mg/L after 48 hours in hospital
   D   Glasgow score > 3
   E   Obesity

3. An 8-week-old infant is diagnosed with a congenital diaphragmatic hernia (CDH).

   What is the most common cause of a CDH?

   A   Anterior defect (Morgagni hernia)
   B   Central tendon defect
   C   Defect in the pleuroperitoneal fold
   D   Enlarged oesophageal hiatus
   E   Posterolateral defect (Morgagni hernia)

4. A 27-year-old man presents with colicky pain in his left flank and urine dipstick reveals the presence of haematuria. A plain abdominal radiograph reveals a 0.5×0.5 cm opacification in his bladder which is thought to represent a passed calculus.

    What is this calculus most likely to be composed of?

    A   Calcium oxalate
    B   Calcium phosphate
    C   Mixed oxalate/phosphate
    D   Ammonium magnesium phosphate (struvite)
    E   Uric acid

5. A 6-year-old boy with abdominal pain is admitted to the paediatric surgical ward for investigation and treatment. He is known from a previous admission to have a Meckel's diverticulum and his attending doctors wonder if it is the cause of his current symptoms.

    Which of the following is not a recognised presentation of a Meckel's diverticulum?

    A   Gastrointestinal haemorrhage
    B   Incidental mesenteric lesion found at laparoscopy/laparotomy
    C   Intussusception
    D   Perforation
    E   Symptomatic inguinal hernia

6. A 3-week-old neonate presents with dehydration and bilious vomiting. A contrast study reveals a duodenojejunal junction lying on the right side of the abdomen.

    What is the most appropriate definitive management?

    A   Hydrostatic reduction
    B   Insertion of nasogastric tube
    C   Intravenous fluids and antiemetics
    D   Laparotomy
    E   Review at 6 months of age to determine the need for intervention

7. A 4-year-old infant is diagnosed with a symptomatic choledochal cyst.

    What is the most appropriate treatment?

    A   Cyst gastrostomy
    B   Cyst jejunostomy
    C   Excision with Roux-en-Y hepaticojejunostomy
    D   Primary excision of the lesion
    E   Surveillance (endoscopic)

8. A 21-year-old previously healthy male arts student presents with a 2-day history of lower abdominal pain and loss of appetite. He is pyrexial and has a tender palpable mass in his right iliac fossa. Haematology reveals a pyogenic leukocytosis and a CT demonstrates a 13 × 15 cm walled-off abscess adjacent to a large complex inflammatory mass involving an inflamed appendix.

What is the most appropriate management plan?

A Conservative management (analgesia, intravenous fluid and antibiotics)
B Conservative management, followed by interval appendicectomy at 6–8 weeks
C Laparoscopy and washout
D Laparoscopic appendicectomy
E Percutaneous drainage of the abscess and intravenous antibiotics

9. A 70-year-old man with arteriopathy undergoes a barium enema and feels light-headed afterwards. Routine biochemistry reveals a serum potassium of 2.8 mmol/L.

Which medication is least likely to be causative?

A Amphotericin B
B Barium
C Furosemide
D Salbutamol
E Trimethoprim

10. A 45-year-old woman with haematemesis is admitted to the emergency department in hypovolaemic shock. She undergoes resuscitation including administration of packed red cells. The blood transfusion centre will not release certain blood products unless a 'massive bleeding' protocol is initiated.

Which of the following is not a definition of massive bleeding?

A Blood loss of half the patient's circulating volume in a 3-hour period
B Blood loss of the patient's circulating volume in a 24-hour period
C Ongoing blood loss of 100 mL/min
D Transfusion of 4 units of red cells in 4 hours with continued bleeding
E Transfusion of 10 units of packed red cells in a 24-hour period

11. A 43-year-old previously well woman presents with pain, swelling and erythema in the anorectal area.

What is the most appropriate management?

A CT of abdomen and pelvis
B Examination under anaesthesia and drainage of pus
C Flexible sigmoidoscopy
D Intravenous antibiotics
E MRI of perineum

12. A 65-year-old man with severe pancreatitis is intubated and ventilated in the intensive care unit. His intra-abdominal pressure is measured using a catheter in his bladder connected to manometry.

Which one of the following describes the pressure effect seen in abdominal compartment syndrome?

   A   Bladder pressure of 16–25 mmHg does not present with oliguria
   B   Bladder pressure of 16–25 mmHg does not require decompression
   C   Bladder pressure of 26–35 mmHg results in increased cardiac output
   D   Bladder pressure of > 35 mmHg does not cause anuria
   E   Bladder pressure of < 15 mmHg normally has clinical signs

13. An 84-year-old man presents repeatedly with abdominal distension due to a sigmoid volvulus.

Which one of the following statements does not apply to the management of sigmoid volvulus?

   A   Following detorsion, volvulus recurs in 50–90% of cases
   B   Following sigmoid resection, volvulus recurs in 0% of cases
   C   Sigmoidoscopic decompression successfully reduces volvulus in 70–80% of cases
   D   Spontaneous detorsion of volvulus is common
   E   Therapeutic barium enema can successfully reduce a volvulus

14. Which of the following is most likely to shift the oxygen haemoglobin dissociation curve to the left?

   A   Decreased pH
   B   Extreme altitude
   C   Increased 2,3-diphosphoglycerate concentration
   D   Increased Paco$_2$
   E   Increased temperature

15. Prothrombin complex concentrate is a haematological product, which is used for patients with ongoing bleeding.

Which of the following statements does not describe prothrombin complex concentrate?

   A   It contains clotting factors II, VII, VIII and IX
   B   It contains protein C and protein S
   C   It has a faster mode of action than fresh frozen plasma
   D   It is used for perioperative prophylaxis of bleeding in acquired deficiency of the prothrombin complex coagulation factors
   E   It is used for reversal of warfarin when rapid correction is required

16. A 22-year-old man sustains a stab wound to the left anterolateral chest wall. He is talking at the scene but on arrival in the emergency department he becomes confused and aggressive and then suffers a cardiac arrest.

Which of the following statements is false?

A   Endotracheal intubation and ventilation should occur prior to resuscitative thoracotomy

B   Isolated cardiac injuries have the best outcome following resuscitative thoracotomy

C   Needle pericardiocentesis in the management of cardiac tamponade is of little value in trauma patients

D   The immediate administration of adrenaline and noradrenaline will improve this patient's chance of survival

E   Thoracic stab wounds have a higher survival rate than thoracic gunshot wounds

17. A 65-year-old man presents with left iliac fossa pain, pyrexia and raised white cell count 20×1000 per mm^3 and C-reactive protein of 200 mg/L.

What is the most appropriate investigation?

A   Abdominal X-ray
B   Barium enema
C   Colonoscopy
D   CT of abdomen and pelvis
E   Flexible sigmoidoscopy

18. A 23-year-old woman is referred by the gastroenterology team with tachycardia, hypotension and generalised colonic tenderness. She has had 5 days of intravenous steroids and her bowel movements have decreased from 12 to 6 bloody stools per day.

What is the most appropriate management?

A   Colonoscopy and biopsies
B   Continue IV steroids
C   Cyclosporin
D   Infliximab
E   Subtotal colectomy and ileostomy

19. A 78-year-old woman is admitted with a dense right-sided weakness. She has reduced consciousness but is moving her left arm and both legs normally. She is confused and disorientated but opens her eyes in response to vocal stimuli and follows commands.

What is this patient's score on the Glasgow Coma Scale?

A   10
B   11
C   12
D   13
E   14

20. ABO compatibility is advisable for the transfusion of blood products.

Which of the following products does not require ABO compatibility?

A   Cryoprecipitate
B   Fresh frozen plasma
C   Haemoglobin solution
D   Packed red cells
E   Platelets

21. A 24-year-old woman is involved in a road traffic accident where she sustains a splenic injury.

Which of the following statements describes the classification of splenic injury?

A   Grade I injury describes an intraparenchymal haematoma <5 cm in diameter
B   Grade II injury describes a capsular tear <1 cm deep
C   Grade III injury describes a subcapsular haematoma <50% of the surface area
D   Grade III injury describes a capsular laceration 1–3 cm deep in the parenchyma
E   Grade IV injury describes a laceration producing major devascularisation (>25% of spleen)

22. A 72-year-old man presents with fresh rectal bleeding. He undergoes CT angiography, which fails to localise the bleeding source and continues to bleed.

What is the most appropriate investigation?

A   Barium enema
B   CT of chest, abdomen and pelvis
C   Colonoscopy
D   Flexible sigmoidoscopy
E   Upper gastrointestinal endoscopy and proctoscopy

23. A 55-year-old man presents to the surgical department with acute colonic bleeding.

Which of the following statements is most appropriate?

A   Angiodysplasia is a rare cause
B   Diverticular bleeding is the most common cause, accounting for approximately 50% of cases
C   For angiography to successfully identify the bleeding source, the blood loss must be above 10 mL/min
D   Rectal causes preclude the need for proximal investigation
E   The incidence of bleeding post polypectomy is as high as 30%

24. A 74-year-old woman attends her GP complaining of absolute constipation and abdominal distension. Her GP is concerned about the possibility of large bowel obstruction.

Which of the following statements describes the features of large bowel obstruction?

A   Colonic volvulus is the most common cause
B   Colonoscopy is the most appropriate first line investigation
C   If the ileocaecal valve is incompetent a closed loop obstruction will develop
D   Nausea and vomiting are early clinical symptoms
E   Signs of peritonitis suggest ischaemia or perforation

25. An 88-year-old woman with severe chronic obstructive pulmonary disease presents with abdominal distension. A CT shows an obstructing apple core lesion of the sigmoid colon. She is also noted to have bilobar liver metastases.

What is the most appropriate first line management?

A   Caecostomy
B   Colonic stenting
C   Hartmann's procedure
D   Sigmoid colectomy
E   Subtotal colectomy and end ileostomy

26. A 72-year-old man with refractory hypotension is commenced on dopamine in the intensive care unit.

Which of the following statements describes dopamine?

A   In high doses it causes peripheral vasodilatation
B   In low doses it increases renal blood flow
C   It decreases cardiac output
D   It decreases splanchnic blood flow
E   It is able to cross the blood–brain barrier

27. A 22-year-old girl has a suspicious lesion on her right shoulder that requires excision biopsy.

Which of the following statements describes the excision margins for malignant skin lesions?

A   In pTis melanoma (in situ) an excision margin of 1 cm is recommended
B   In pT1 melanoma (0–1 mm thickness) an excision margin of 2 cm is recommended
C   In pT4 melanoma (>4 mm thickness) an excision margin of 2 cm is recommended
D   With primary basal cell carcinoma lesions <2 cm in diameter, an excision margin of 0.5–1.0 cm is recommended
E   With squamous cell carcinoma lesions <2 cm, a margin of 1 cm is recommended

28. A 60-year-old man presents with large volume haematemesis. After resuscitation an endoscopy reveals bleeding varices in the fundus of the stomach with no other abnormalities seen.

What is the most appropriate initial treatment?

A   Balloon tamponade
B   Band ligation
C   Blood pressure regulation
D   Injection of cyanoacrylate glue
E   Transjugular intrahepatic portosystemic shunt

29. A 66-year-old man has long-standing portal hypertension due to alcohol abuse. He is investigated on an outpatient basis for the development of varices.

Which of the following anatomical areas does not represent a site of portosystemic varices?

A   Intrahepatic, between the portal vein and the inferior vena cava
B   Lower oesophagus, between the left gastric vein and oesophageal branches of the azygous vein
C   Rectal, between the superior rectal vein and the pudendal vein
D   Retroperitoneal, between the ovarian vessels and the renal veins
E   Umbilical, between the obliterated umbilical vein and the left portal vein

30. Which of the following pathogens are not eradicated by alcohol-based hand gels?

A   *Clostridium difficile*
B   *Escherichia coli*
C   Extended spectrum β-lactamase
D   *Klebsiella* species
E   Methicillin-resistant *Staphylococcus aureus*

31. A 47-year-old woman presents to the emergency department with generalised weakness, fatigue and light headedness. Her routine blood gases show: pH 7.34, Pao_2 9.4 kPa, $Paco_2$ 4.4 kPa, HCO_3 22 mmol/L. Serum biochemistry includes Na^+ 131 mmol/L, K^+ 5.1 mmol/L, and plasma glucose 3.4 mmol/L.

What is the most likely diagnosis?

A   Addison's disease
B   Chronic renal failure
C   Diabetic ketoacidosis
D   Exacerbation of chronic obstructive pulmonary disease
E   Myasthenia gravis

32. A 47-year-old man has an open appendicectomy. A 2.5 cm carcinoid tumour with clear resection margins is diagnosed on histopathology.

What is the most appropriate management?

A Chemotherapy
B Colonoscopy
C No further management required
D Right hemicolectomy
E Subtotal colectomy and ileorectal anastomosis

33. A study is performed to assess whether there is a correlation between the time a patient waits for colonoscopy (irrespective of outcome) and the overall satisfaction rating for the in-hospital experience. Waiting time is divided into four ascending groups and satisfaction is scored on a continuous rating scale from 1 to 100.

Which statistical test should be used to examine for any association?

A ANOVA test
B Kruskal–Wallis test
C Linear regression analysis
D Mann–Whitney U test
E Two-sided *t*-test

34. A controlled study is set up to address whether or not patients having single incision laparoscopic cholecystectomy have similar outcomes to standard laparoscopic cholecystectomy. The primary outcome measure is complication rate, estimated at 5% for the standard procedure. To detect a difference of 2.5%, in either direction, it is decided that 200 patients require to be recruited to both arms of the study, with a power of 80%.

Which statement best describes the application of statistical principles?

A A significant difference (*p*-value = 0.05) has a likelihood of being due to chance in 1 in 20 cases
B All patients should be offered either procedure by the clinician
C If early results show inferiority, the trial continues to allow conclusions to be drawn
D If there is low recruitment, there is a risk of a type I error
E The study will be underpowered to detect this difference

35. A surgeon would like to know whether patients with thyroid goitres are more or less likely to have been exposed to irradiation during their early years, than those patients without goitres.

What is the best study design for this purpose?

A   Case–control study
B   Environmental study
C   Longitudinal cohort study
D   Meta-analysis of the literature
E   Randomised trial of exposure

36. A surgeon would like to set up a randomised double-blind controlled trial, examining the efficacy of laparoscopic fundoplication (comparing partial and total wrap). The outcomes are defined and a power calculation performed, and the centre is ready to start recruitment.

Which factor is not essential to the validity of the trial?

A   Adopting a recognised method for patient allocation and stratification
B   Blinding the patients
C   Blinding the surgical team
D   Ensuring it represents a more general population
E   Having randomisation conducted through a remote site

37. A 95-year-old man is admitted from a nursing home with diarrhoea and is subsequently diagnosed with colitis secondary to *Clostridium difficile.*

Which of the following statements describes *Clostridium difficile* infection?

A   Cephalosporins are rarely associated with the diagnosis
B   First line medical therapy is intravenous metronidazole
C   Its presentation is consistently more severe than other forms of gastroenteritis
D   Patients with prolonged hospital stays are at particular risk
E   Vancomycin is a frequent risk factor

38. A 22-year-old girl is admitted with collapse and dehydration. She is suspected of being chronically malnourished.

Which of the following statements describes malnutrition assessment in the acute hospital setting?

A   Every malnourished patient should have trace elements checked prior to commencing on supplements
B   Formal diagnosis of malnutrition may be made with body mass index (BMI) $\leq 18\,\text{kg/m}^2$
C   Obese patients do not require nutritional screening
D   Only patients with clinical or biochemical signs of malnutrition require nutritional screening at admission
E   The Malnutrition Universal Screening Tool calculates risk by patient's reduction in BMI

39. Which of the following statements does not describe evidence based medicine?

   A   Absolute risk reduction: effect of an intervention minus effect observed in controls

   B   Number needed to treat: effectiveness of an intervention (equivalent to 1 ÷ absolute risk reduction).

   C   Odds ratio: likelihood of being exposed to a risk factor

   D   Prevalence: risk of developing a new condition within a specified period

   E   Relative risk: likelihood of an outcome, relative to an exposure status

40. A 70-year-old woman is receiving peripheral total parenteral nutrition (TPN) following an emergency laparotomy for small bowel obstruction. The cannula tissues and the TPN extravasates.

Which is the most appropriate treatment:

   A   Apply a cold compress and elevate the limb

   B   Phentolamine

   C   Hyaluronidase

   D   Ascorbic acid injection

   E   Hydrocortisone sodium succinate

41. A 22-year-old boy is seriously injured in a road traffic accident and following discussion with his family, is being considered as an organ donor.

Which of the following is not a precondition for the diagnosis of brainstem death?

   A   A $Paco_2$ of >7 kPa has been documented

   B   All underlying metabolic or pharmacological causes have been excluded

   C   If neuromuscular blockade has been administered, a return to normal state has been demonstrated

   D   Tests are performed by two doctors trained in the technique on two separate occasions

   E   There is no papillary reflex to light (cranial nerves II and III)

42. Which of the following statements describes the limitations of day case surgery?

   A   Diabetic patients can easily be managed on a day case list

   B   Obese patients (BMI >30) should be excluded from day case lists

   C   Patients must have a responsible carer accompanying them for 24–48 hours postoperatively

   D   Patients must have a telephone in the discharge destination

   E   The procedure should have a low incidence of postoperative complications

43. A 3-week-old neonate presents with crying and vomiting and malrotation is suspected.

Which of the following statements describes malrotation of the gut?

A The caecum fails to descend to a subhepatic position during embryological development

B It is frequently associated with other congenital abnormalities

C The diagnosis is based on is bilious vomiting in the first few days of life

D There is normal gas pattern on plain X-ray and the diagnosis requires a contrast study

E With neonatal bilious vomiting, definitive surgery may be deferred until nutritional issues are addressed

44. A 4-year-old infant presents with the passage of 'redcurrant' stool. The paediatric surgeons are suspicious of intussusception.

Which of the following statements describes intussusception in the paediatric population?

A At operation a resection of the affected bowel is always required

B It is caused by a congenital anatomical variant

C It can be treated by air enema without risk

D It most commonly affects the 4- to 6-year-old age group

E It most commonly occurs in an ileocolic segment of bowel

45. A 15-year-old boy is involved in a fight and sustains a stab wound to his right upper quadrant/epigastrium. On presentation to the emergency department he is lucid, oxygenating, but complaining of abdominal pain, with a systolic blood pressure of 90 mmHg, on his second litre of crystalloid. On examination, he has peritonitis and his blood pressure is not stabilising.

What is the most appropriate next step in the management plan?

A CT of the abdomen to delineate injuries

B Focused assessment with sonography for trauma scan to confirm fluid/gas in the peritoneal cavity

C Laparotomy in emergency theatre

D Serum amylase level

E Urinary catheter insertion

46. A 2-year-old boy presents with painless bleeding per rectum. He is diagnosed with a bleeding Meckel's diverticulum.

Which of the following statements is true?

A CT angiogram is the imaging investigation of choice

B Cimetidine decreases diagnostic yield of imaging techniques

C Meckel's diverticulum is caused by complete obliteration of the vitelline duct

D The vitelline duct should close by 12 weeks' duration

E The blood supply of a Meckel's diverticulum is from the omphalomesenteric artery

47. Which of the following statements describes pyloric stenosis?

    A   Bilious vomiting is frequently associated with the diagnosis
    B   In >50% cases, it presents in the first 2 weeks of life
    C   Infants present with a hypochloraemic, hypokalaemic metabolic alkalosis
    D   It most commonly presents in first born female infants
    E   Surgical correction must take place within the first 24 hours of presentation

48. A 5-year-old child with pain in his right iliac fossa is suspected to have acute appendicitis.

Which of the following statements describes appendicitis in children?

    A   A child with peritonitis should have volume resuscitation (≥ 20 mL/kg intravenous fluid) prior to surgery
    B   Diagnosis is easier to reach than in adults, and tends to present at an earlier stage
    C   Elevated white cell count and C-reactive protein are prerequisites before taking the child to theatre
    D   Laparoscopic appendicectomy is contraindicated in children under 6 years of age
    E   Signs are ordinarily specific, but diagnosis is aided by sequential re-examination

49. A 31-year-old farmer is shot in the abdomen. He is taken to hospital and a damage control laparotomy is performed.

Which of the following statements best describes damage control surgery?

    A   Only the abdomen should be prepped to avoid unnecessary exposure and hypothermia
    B   Diagnostic tests should be utilised prior to theatre to ensure a complete injury profile is known
    C   Laparotomy may result in loss of intra-abdominal tamponade and therefore should be avoided
    D   Medial visceral rotation manoeuvres may be required to fully inspect the retroperitoneum
    E   Angiographic embolisation is not required if a thorough damage control laparotomy has been performed

50. A 44-year-old woman falls from a significant height and sustains injuries to her head and torso.

Which of the following is a component of the secondary survey as per the Advanced Trauma Life Support (ATLS) protocol?

    A   Alert, voice, pain unresponsive assessment of neurological status
    B   Control of haemorrhage
    C   Focused assessment with sonography for trauma scan
    D   Log roll including checking spinal integrity and anal tone
    E   Respiratory rate

51. A 19-year-old man presents to resuscitation in the emergency department following a high-energy, two-vehicle, head-on road traffic accident. He was unrestrained in the front passenger seat. At primary survey, his airway appears patent, but he is alert only to painful stimuli, and his oxygen saturations are falling below 92% on non-rebreathing mask. There is a possibility of pulmonary contusions. He is also noted to have significant maxillary swelling and bruising. There is no apparent circulatory compromise.

What is the next priority in the management plan?

A   Airway management – Guedel airway
B   Airway management – nasopharyngeal airway
C   Airway management – needle cricothyroidotomy
D   Airway management – prepare for definitive orotracheal airway and have surgical airway kit ready
E   Breathing management – two-person bag valve mask

52. A patient with gastric cancer is undergoing preoperative work up. He completes cardiopulmonary exercise testing (CPEX).

Which one of the following statements is true?

A   A measurement of carbon dioxide consumption is undertaken
B   Recent myocardial infarction does not preclude testing
C   Patients are advised to drink caffeine 30 minutes prior to testing
D VO_2 at anaerobic threshold of >8 mL/kg/min is a predictor of low cardiovascular risk after major abdominal surgery
E   Written consent must be taken prior to commencing CPEX

53. Which of the following statements describes the features of inotropic agents?

A   Adrenaline is frequently the agent of choice in cardiogenic shock
B   Dopamine acts primarily on β_2-adrenoceptors with positive inotropic and chronotropic effects
C   Glyceryl trinitrate is a useful additive agent in cardiac failure to decrease the afterload
D   Noradrenaline is frequently the agent of choice in septic shock
E   Use of dopexamine may compromise the splanchnic circulation through positive β_2-agonism

54. Which of the following physiological abnormalities is not caused by massive transfusion?

A   Acidaemia
B   Coagulopathy
C   Hyperkalaemia
D   Hyperthermia
E   Hypomagnesaemia

55. Which of the following statements describes systemic inflammatory response syndrome (SIRS)?

   A   A heart rate of > 90 beats per minute and a respiratory rate of > 20 breaths per minute are adequate diagnostic criteria for SIRS

   B   At least single organ failure is present in SIRS

   C   Disseminated intravascular coagulation and related bleeding problems are characteristic of SIRS

   D   The diagnosis of SIRS requires the presence of a bacteraemia

   E   Vasoconstriction is the prominent cardiovascular response

56. Which of the following statements describes mechanical ventilation?

   A   It is usually beneficial to acute kidney injury

   B   It can be used to aid raised intracranial pressure by increasing intrathoracic pressure

   C   It must always be instigated when $Pao_2 > 8$ kPa

   D   Reduced blood pressure and cardiac output is an important side effect

   E   There is an increase in the patient's own response to trauma and metabolic drive

57. A 65-year-old man falls 2 m from a ladder. He sustains blunt thoracic trauma.

   Which of the following statements is correct?

   A   Flail chest is defined radiographically as three or more consecutive ribs fractured in two or more places

   B   Open reduction and internal fixation of rib fractures is only of benefit in flail chest

   C   In blunt thoracic trauma rib fractures usually occur in isolation

   D   Patients with flail chest should be managed with intubation and positive pressure ventilation

   E   Nonunion of rib fractures should be managed conservatively

58. A 47-year-old man is brought to the emergency department having been trapped in a burning house for 20 minutes before rescue. He has sustained burns to his entire back, and left arm, anteriorly and posteriorly and they are red and painful. He does not appear to have airway compromise, and in particular there is no singing of nasal hairs. His blood pressure and pulse are acceptable. His estimated weight is 80 kg.

   What is the most appropriate resuscitation plan?

   A   3 L compound crystalloid over 8 hours, and the same again over the next 16 hours

   B   4.5 L compound crystalloid over 8 hours, and the same again over the next 16 hours

   C   4.5 L compound crystalloid over 12 hours, and the same again over the next 12 hours

   D   8.5 L compound crystalloid over 12 hours

   E   Bolus resuscitation with colloid until urinary output established

59. An intensive care unit is a specially staffed and equipped, separate and self-contained area of a hospital dedicated to the management and monitoring of patients with life-threatening conditions.

Which of the following statements regarding intensive care facilities is true?

A   Consultant-to-patient ratio should be between 1:2 and 1:8
B   Intensive care units provide level 1 care
C   Admission to the intensive care unit should take place within 30 minutes of the decision to admit
D   All intensive care units must have the facility to provide extracorporeal membrane oxygenation
E   Night-time discharge from the intensive care unit is associated with poorer patient outcomes

60. A 72-year-old man with a previous history of deep vein thrombosis undergoes a straightforward anterior resection with primary anastomosis for a high rectal carcinoma. At postoperative day 4, he appears ready to go home, but complains of a swollen, tender right leg. He is diagnosed with a deep vein thrombosis, commencing therapeutic dose low-molecular weight heparin immediately, with a plan for warfarinisation. That night, he becomes acutely unwell, with dyspnoea, abdominal pain and distension, and high fever. Free gas is seen on his chest X-ray. Following instigation of intravenous fluids and antibiotics, what is the most appropriate next step in the management plan?

A   Conservative management of anastomotic leak with further fluids, antibiotics, +/– radiological drain and commence warfarinisation
B   Conservative management of anastomotic leak with further fluids, antibiotics, +/– radiological drain and continue to administer heparin
C   Placement of a caval filter prior to return to theatre for anastomotic leak
D   Return to theatre for anastomotic leak
E   Reversal of heparin prior to return to theatre for anastomotic leak

61. A 63-year-old diabetic man is admitted as an emergency to the surgical ward and diagnosed with idiopathic, acute severe pancreatitis. He rapidly deteriorates, with a need for ventilatory support, and his oliguria evolves into anuria within 48 hours. He is obese, but his abdomen is distended and tender, with apparent diaphragmatic splinting. His arterial gas pattern shows a mild metabolic acidaemia, with a Pao_2 of 7.8 kPa and $Paco_2$ of 6.0 kPa on 80% Fio_2. Non-invasive ventilation is considered, and he requires renal haemofiltration.

What is the most likely diagnosis?

A   Abdominal compartment syndrome
B   Acute kidney injury
C   Established renal failure
D   Necrotic pancreatitis
E   Type 2 respiratory failure

Questions: EMIs

Theme: Small bowel obstruction

A	Adhesions	G	Incisional hernia
B	Bezoar	H	Inguinal hernia
C	Caecal carcinoma	I	Postoperative ileus
D	Diaphragmatic hernia	J	Pseudomyxoma peritonei
E	Femoral hernia	K	Recurrent Crohn's disease
F	Gallstone ileus	L	Small bowel tumour

Instructions: For each of the following scenarios, choose the single most likely pathology from the list above. Each option may be used once, more than once or not at all.

62. A 45-year-old woman with Crohn's disease develops sudden onset bilious vomiting and abdominal distension. Her history includes a previous right hemicolectomy for terminal ileal disease 15 years ago with two further small bowel resections.

63. A 78-year-old woman describes recent vague upper abdominal pain and now has profuse vomiting. Erect chest X-ray demonstrates an unusual gas pattern in the right upper quadrant and abdominal X-ray shows dilated small bowel loops proximal to an opacification in the right lower quadrant.

64. A 35-year-old man with cachexia, lower abdominal pain and vomiting undergoes laparoscopy for planned appendicectomy. After encountering difficulties creating a pneumoperitoneum there is very poor visibility because of gelatinous material in the peritoneal cavity.

Theme: Statistical testing

A	Analysis of variance (ANOVA)	G	Mann–Whitney U test
B	χ^2 test	H	Multivariate analysis
C	Friedman's test	I	Paired t-test
D	Independent t-test	J	Pearson's correlation coefficient
E	Kruskal–Wallis	K	Spearman's rank correlation
F	Kaplan–Meier	L	Wilcoxon signed-rank testing

Instructions: For each of the following descriptions, choose the single most appropriate statistical test from the list above. Each option may be used once, more than once or not at all.

65. A test for comparison of proportions.

66. A non-parametric test for comparison of central location between two independent samples.

67. A non-parametric test for evaluating the difference between several related samples.

Theme: Investigation of operative complications

A   Abdominal radiograph
B   Abdominal ultrasound
C   Arterial blood gases
D   Barium enema
E   Blood cultures
F   Chest radiograph
G   CT of the chest

H   CT of the abdomen
I   Gastrografin enema
J   Laparoscopy
K   Laparotomy
L   Urine culture
M   Wound swab

Instructions: For each of the following scenarios, choose the single most appropriate investigation from the list above. Each option may be used once, more than once or not at all.

68. A 48-year-old woman has an uneventful laparoscopic cholecystectomy for symptomatic gallstones. 6 days following surgery she represents complaining of upper abdominal pain and distension.

69. A 78-year-old man undergoes a Lichtenstein repair of a painful left inguinal hernia. 3 weeks later, he complains of gradual onset left lower quadrant pain and tenderness. He has a past medical history of chronic obstructive pulmonary disease, diverticular disease and type 2 diabetes.

70. An 81-year-old man undergoes an anterior resection with primary anastomosis for a T3 N1 carcinoma of his mid-rectum. On the sixth postoperative day he has an ongoing ileus with diffuse lower abdominal pain. He has a mild fever at $37.6°C$ and abdominal examination reveals fullness in the left iliac fossa which is tender. There is a leukocytosis of 15×1000 per mm^3.

Theme: Miscellaneous herniae

A   Amyand's
B   Diaphragmatic
C   Femoral
D   Incisional
E   Lanz
F   Littre's
G   Maydl's

H   Pantaloon
I   Paraumbilical
J   Petit's
K   Richter's
L   Spigelian
M   Umbilical

Instructions: For each of the following scenarios, choose the single most appropriate term from the list above. Each option may be used once, more than once or not at all.

71. An 85-year-old man undergoes open surgical repair of a symptomatic hernia. During the operation the hernial sac is found to contain an inflamed appendix.

72. A 45-year-old man has two adjacent loops of small bowel that are located within a hernial sac with a tight neck. The portion of bowel in-between is deprived of its blood supply and is progressing towards necrosis.

73. A 70-year-old obese woman has a right-sided swelling due to a combination of direct and indirect hernia. At operation the hernial sacs bulge on either side of the inferior epigastric vessels.

Theme: Hepatitis and blood-borne viruses

A   Hepatitis C virus (HVC) polymerase chain reaction (PCR)
B   Hepatitis B core antibody
C   Hepatitis B DNA
D   Hepatitis B e antibody
E   Hepatitis B e antigen
F   Hepatitis B IgM core antibody
G   Hepatitis B surface antibody
H   Hepatitis B surface antigen
I   Hepatitis C antibody
J   HIV type 1 serology
K   HIV type 2 serology
L   Human T-lymphotropic virus serology

Instructions: For each of the following descriptions, choose the single most appropriate test from the list above. Each option may be used once, more than once or not at all.

74. A baseline diagnostic test to differentiate between ongoing or resolved hepatitis B in unwell patients. This test is used to determine the transmissibility of hepatitis B.

75. A test to assess response to immunisation in healthcare workers.

76. A test used by specialists to monitor hepatitis C treatment.

Theme: Investigation and treatment of acute biliary pathology

A   CT
B   Diagnostic endoscopic retrograde cholangiopancreatography (ERCP)
C   Endoscopic ultrasound
D   ERCP with balloon trawl with or without sphincterotomy
E   Fine-needle aspiration
F   Laparoscopic cholecystectomy alone
G   Laparoscopic cholecystectomy with on-table cholangiogram
H   Laparoscopic cholecystectomy with bile duct exploration
I   Lithotripsy
J   Magnetic resonance cholangiopancreatography (MRCP)
K   Percutaneous transhepatic cholangiography (PTC)
L   Ursodeoxycholic acid
M   Ultrasound

Instructions: For each of the following scenarios, choose the single most appropriate investigation from the list above. Each option may be used once, more than once or not at all.

77. A 58-year-old woman represents with recurrent upper abdominal pain. She has had a recent abdominal ultrasound which demonstrated stones in the gallbladder with no ductal abnormality. She is apyrexial with normal inflammatory markers, but her liver function tests are grossly abnormal.

78. A 44-year-old woman presents with constant right upper quadrant pain and pyrexia. An ultrasound scan shows a thickened gallbladder containing sludge and a common bile duct (CBD) diameter of 15 mm. No ductal stones are identified but there are poor views of the distal CBD.

79. A 64-year-old man is admitted as an emergency with minor severity gallstone pancreatitis. An abdominal ultrasound scan confirms pancreatitis with gallstones in the gallbladder. There is no duct dilatation.

Theme: Anal and perianal conditions

A	Anal carcinoma	H	Pilonidal sinus
B	Anal fissure	I	Proctalgia fugax
C	Fistula-in-ano	J	Proctitis
D	Ischiorectal abscess	K	Prolapsed thrombosed haemorrhoid
E	Perianal abscess	L	Rectal carcinoma
F	Perianal Crohn's	M	Solitary rectal ulcer syndrome
G	Perianal haematoma	N	Tuberculosis

Instructions: For each of the following scenarios, choose the single most likely diagnosis from the list above. Each option may be used once, more than once or not at all.

80. A 29-year-old woman complains of perianal pain. She describes occasional bleeding and discharge from a midline opening which is 6 cm posterior to the anal verge in natal cleft.

81. A 54-year-old man has pain after defaecation and has also noticed blood on the toilet paper.

82. A 44-year-old woman has noticed the discharge of foul smelling fluid from lateral to the anal verge. She has a visible pit in the midline.

Theme: Scrotal conditions

A	Epididymo-orchitis	H	Inguinoscrotal hernia
B	Epididymal cyst	I	Seminoma
C	Epididymitis	J	Teratoma
D	Haematoma	K	Testicular torsion
E	Hydrocoele	L	Torsion of the hydatid of Morgagni
F	Idiopathic scrotal oedema	M	Varicocele
G	Idiopathic scrotal haemorrhage		

Instructions: For each of the following scenarios, choose the single most likely diagnosis from the list above. Each option may be used once, more than once or not at all.

83. A 32-year-old man is struck in the groin by a football and on self-examining he notices a painless non-tender 1.5 cm swelling on his left testicle. His GP takes some blood tests and identifies a raised serum β-hCG and α-fetoprotein.

84. A 27-year-old man has a painless 2 cm swelling in the upper pole of his right testicle. It transilluminates and is palpable separate from the testis.

85. A 4-year-old infant has painless non-tender bilateral scrotal swelling. He has an erythematous area extending towards his perineum.

Theme: Management of scrotal swellings

A Analgesia and close observation
B Antibiotics
C Aspiration
D Excision of cyst
E Herniotomy
F Immediate surgical exploration

G Jaboulay procedure
H Liechtenstein repair of inguinal hernia
I Ligation of left testicular vein
J Lord's procedure
K Testicular vein embolisation

Instructions: For each of the following scenarios, choose the single most appropriate treatment from the list above. Each option may be used once, more than once or not at all.

86. A 32-year-old man has a cystic swelling on the upper pole of his right testicle, which he finds uncomfortable when cycling to work.

87. A 17-year-old has a 5-hour history of severe pain in his right testicle. It is tender and lying high in the scrotum.

88. A 37-year-old man has an asymptomatic swelling in his left testicle. He describes it as 'a bag of worms' and on standing there is a noticeable increase in size.

Theme: Right iliac fossa pain

A Appendicitis
B Appendix mass
C Caecal carcinoma
D Diverticular disease
E Ectopic pregnancy
F Mesenteric adenitis
G Mittelschmerz

H Pelvic inflammatory disease
I Perforated viscus
J Renal colic
K Ruptured ovarian cyst
L Terminal ileal Crohn's disease
M Urinary tract infection

Instructions: For each of the following scenarios, choose the single most likely diagnosis from the list above. Each option may be used once, more than once or not at all.

89. A 29-year-old woman presents with a 2-day history of right iliac fossa pain. It was fairly sudden in onset and radiates through to her back. She has no bowel or urinary symptoms and it is 2 weeks since her last period. Ultrasound scan reveals a trace of fluid in the pelvis but no other abnormalities.

90. An 8-year-old boy complains of a 2-day history of right iliac fossa pain. He is apyrexial but is guarding with rebound tenderness. He has had a runny nose for the past few days and despite his pain he is hungry and very thirsty. There is a strong family history of inflammatory bowel disease.

91. A 39-year-old man presents with a 4-week history of feeling generally unwell. He has low grade pyrexia and is off his food. His clothes feel looser and he suspects he has lost nearly 10 kg. He has not vomited but has been diarrhoeal up to 10 times per day. He is tender in the right iliac fossa, where there is a palpable mass.

Theme: Investigation and management of trauma

A   Chest radiograph
B   CT of chest, abdomen and pelvis
C   CT of head
D   Decompression of tension
     pneumothorax
E   Diagnostic peritoneal lavage
F   Intercostal chest drain

G   Intravenous access and fluid
     resuscitation
H   Laparotomy
I   Pericardiocentesis
J   Skull radiograph
K   Thoracotomy
L   Ultrasound of the abdomen

Instructions: For each of the following scenarios, choose the single most appropriate intervention from the list above. Each option may be used once, more than once or not at all.

92. A 62-year-old man is the restrained driver in a head-on collision with another car at approximately 50 miles per hour. He complains of right-sided chest and thigh pain. He is alert but uncooperative with multiple superficial grazes. His pulse is 140 beats per minute, blood pressure is 100/74 mmHg. His trachea is deviated to the left and he has a hyperresonant right hemithorax. His abdomen is soft but there is some bruising in the right upper quadrant.

93. A 27-year-old man is brought to the emergency department resuscitation room following a high-speed road traffic accident. He is in asystole and a focused assessment with sonography for trauma (FAST) scan suggests a pericardial effusion and some free fluid in the abdomen. Pericardiocentesis is performed and a small volume of blood is aspirated. His clinical condition does not improve. He is also noticed to have a tense abdomen.

94. A 45-year-old male intravenous drug abuser is stabbed in the epigastric region with a breadknife. On arrival to the emergency department, he is hypotensive with a thread pulse of 160 beats per minute. His SpO_2 is maintained at 95% on 15 L 100% O_2 and he has two large-bore Venflon catheters inserted with fast resuscitation fluid. There is a 3 cm incision midway between his umbilicus and xiphisternum with visible omentum. During FAST scanning, he deteriorates and becomes haemodynamically unstable.

Theme: Scoring systems

A	1		G	7
B	2		H	8
C	3		I	9
D	4		J	10
E	5		K	11
F	6			

Instructions: For each of the following scenarios, choose the single most likely numerical score from the list above. Each option may be used once, more than once or not at all.

95. A 60-year-old man with liver disease is assessed using the Child–Pugh score. His bilirubin is 44 µmol/L. The International normalised ratio is 1.0 and albumin is 40 g/L. He has no ascites or hepatic encephalopathy.

96. A 52-year-old man with acute pancreatitis is assessed during his first 48 hours in hospital. His modified Glasgow acute pancreatitis score is calculated. His arterial blood gas on air is normal. His serum urea is 15.6 mmol/L and his white cell count is 17.8×10^9/L. There rest of his blood tests are normal.

97. A 64-year-old man is admitted with melaena and haematemesis. His past medical history includes ischaemic heart disease and type 2 diabetes. At presentation he is clammy with a tachycardia of 120 beats per minute and his blood pressure is 92/58 mmHg. He undergoes urgent endoscopy which identifies a Mallory–Weiss tear which has stopped bleeding. His risk of further bleeding and an adverse outcome is assessed using the Rockall score.

Theme: Skin lesions

A	Acanthosis nigricans	H	Keratoacanthoma
B	Basal cell carcinoma	I	Nodular melanoma
C	Calciphylaxis	J	Seborrhoeic keratosis
D	Dermatomyositis (lung cancer)	K	Squamous cell carcinoma
E	Intradermal naevus	L	Strawberry naevus
F	Junctional naevus	M	Thrombophlebitis migrans
G	Lentigo maligna		

Instructions: For each of the following scenarios, choose the single most likely diagnosis from the list above. Each option may be used once, more than once or not at all.

98. A 58-year-old man with stage 5 chronic kidney disease develops painful purple skin lesions with small areas of necrosis on both shins. All pedal pulses are present and there is no venous incompetence.

99. A 45-year-old man is diagnosed with stomach cancer and he is also noted to have dark thickened skin in several of his body folds and creases.

100. A 69-year-old woman describes a discoloured patch on her left cheek, which she has not noticed any change in approximately 15 years. It has an irregular border and is thickened and pigmented with central nodularity.

Theme: Cardiac medication

A	Adenosine	H	Dobutamine
B	Adrenaline	I	Dopamine
C	Amiloride	J	Furosemide
D	Aspirin	K	Metolazone
E	Atenolol	L	Noradrenaline
F	Bendroflumethiazide	M	Simvastatin
G	Digoxin		

Instructions: For each of the following descriptions, choose the single most appropriate medication from the list above. Each option may be used once, more than once or not at all.

101. A weak diuretic associated with hyperkalaemia.

102. A medication which is absolutely contraindicated in pregnancy.

103. A sympathomimetic with mainly α-adrenergic activity.

Theme: Tumour markers

A	5-Hydroxyindoleacetic acid	I	Carcinoembryonic antigen
B	α-Fetoprotein	J	Human epidermal growth factor receptor 2 (HER-2)
C	Bence Jones protein		
D	Cancer antigen (CA) 15-3	K	Lactate dehydrogenase
E	Cancer antigen (CA) 19-9	L	Prostate specific antigen
F	Cancer antigen (CA) 27.29	M	Human chorionic gonadotrophin
G	Cancer antigen (CA) 125	N	Thyroglobulin
H	Calcitonin		

Instructions: For each of the following scenarios, choose the single most likely tumour marker from the list above. Each option may be used once, more than once or not at all.

104. A 48-year-old woman has recently undergone treatment for hepatocellular carcinoma and a tumour marker is used to assess her response to treatment.

105. A 62-year-old woman with obstructive jaundice has an elevated marker for pancreatic cancer.

106. A 23-year-old man with a painless left testicular swelling has an urgent review where tumour markers are taken. One of these is strongly positive and he is diagnosed with a pure seminoma.

Theme: Neonatal pathology

A	Duodenal atresia	G	Malrotation
B	Duplication cyst	H	Meckel's diverticulum
C	Exomphalos	I	Meconium ileus
D	Gastroschisis	J	Necrotising enterocolitis
E	Hirschsprung's disease	K	Pyloric stenosis
F	Intussusception	L	Tracheo-oesophageal fistula

Instructions: For each of the following scenarios, choose the single most likely diagnosis from the list above. Each option may be used once, more than once or not at all.

107. A newborn term boy with a prenatal diagnosis of Down's syndrome has profuse bilious vomiting. There is a double bubble gas pattern on plain abdominal X-ray.

108. A newborn girl with suspected cystic fibrosis has abdominal distension and bilious vomiting.

109. A 2-day-old neonate has been vomiting for approximately 12 hours. She has not passed any meconium since delivery. After insertion of a finger into the rectum, there is an explosive release of gas and diarrhoea.

Theme: Statistical terms

A	Coefficient of variation	H	p-value
B	Confidence interval	I	Positive predictive value
C	Forest plot	J	Power
D	Funnel plot	K	Sensitivity
E	Histogram	L	Specificity
F	Likelihood ratio	M	Standard deviation
G	Negative predictive value	N	Standard error

Instructions: For each of the following descriptions, choose the single most appropriate statistical term from the list above. Each option may be used once, more than once or not at all.

110. A visual method used in meta-analysis to demonstrate the relative strength of treatment effects in scientific studies examining the same question.

111. The chance of developing a type I error.

112. A measure used to compare the ratio of whether a given test result would be expected in a patient with the target disorder under investigation, compared to the chance the same result would be expected in a patient without the target disorder.

Theme: Study design

A   Case–control study
B   Case report
C   Environmental exposure study
D   Feasibility trial of intervention
E   Longitudinal cohort series
F   Meta-analysis
G   Nested case–control trial
H   Randomised controlled trial
I   Systematic review

Instructions: For each of the following scenarios, choose the single most appropriate test from the list above. Each option may be used once, more than once or not at all.

113. A surgeon hypothesises that patients presenting with incisional hernias from laparotomy wounds at 1 year postoperative are more likely to have body mass index > 25.

114. A research registrar is increasingly convinced that laparoscopic colonic resections are yielding improved patient outcomes in terms of length of stay and pain scores. He is aware of a number of studies which have reported these outcomes. He would like to mathematically model the cumulative outcomes data.

115. A young consultant is appointed to establish laparoscopic hepatic resection service in his hospital. After 3 years, he has meticulous data to demonstrate patient risk factors and favourable surgical outcomes. He wishes to write up his work.

Theme: Statistical tests

A χ^2 test
B   Fisher's exact test
C   Kruskal–Wallis test
D   Linear regression
E   Mann–Whitney U test
F   McNemar test
G   Multi-logistic regression
H   Student's t-test
I   Wilcoxon sign rank test

Instructions: For each of the following scenarios, choose the single most appropriate test from the list above. Each option may be used once, more than once or not at all.

116. A surgeon has been gathering data on laparoscopic cholecystectomy (patient details and outcomes) for a number of years. He would like to know if men or women are more likely to have had readmissions with specific complications postoperatively. He has approximately 300 patients on his database.

117. A colorectal surgeon is interested in technology appraisal and wants to define the effectiveness of his own practice, comparing open and laparoscopic approaches for malignant disease. He chooses lymph node yield as a comparative outcome measure.

118. A surgeon believes that patients' pain following inguinal hernia repair is dependent on the mode of surgery (open under general anaesthetic, open under local anaesthetic, transabdominal preperitoneal or total extraperitoneal laparoscopic techniques). The other surgeons in his unit agree to share their patient data, of which there are good numbers for comparisons. Standard postoperative pain scores (0–10) have been collated for every patient prior to discharge.

Theme: Facial nerve palsy

A	Acoustic neuroma	F	Idiopathic (Bell's palsy)
B	Basal skull fracture	G	Previous pleomorphic adenoma
C	Cerebrovascular accident	H	Ramsay Hunt syndrome
D	Chronic otitis media	I	Squamous cell carcinoma
E	Facial trauma		

Instructions: For each of the following scenarios, choose the single most likely diagnosis from the list above. Each option may be used once, more than once or not at all.

119. A 43-year-old alcoholic man has a right-sided palsy and some associated hearing loss. He has been involved in a variety of alcohol-related traumas over the years.

120. A 28-year-old woman undergoing chemotherapy for Hodgkin's lymphoma develops a painful rash around her ear prior to noticing unilateral facial drooping and loss of taste.

121. A 62-year-old man, who has been a heavy smoker and drinker, previously treated for cancer of the tongue presents with discharge from his ear in combination with a left sided facial palsy.

Theme: Superficial skin lesions

A	Basal cell carcinoma	F	Malignant melanoma
B	Dermatofibroma	G	Pyogenic granuloma
C	Dermoid cyst	H	Senile keratosis
D	Keratoacanthoma	I	Squamous cell carcinoma
E	Lentigo maligna		

Instructions: For each of the following scenarios, choose the single most likely diagnosis from the list above. Each option may be used once, more than once or not at all.

122. A 32-year-old woman presents to her GP, concerned about the sudden appearance of a uniform, raised, pigmented lesion on her shin. It has appeared in the last fortnight, and she has recently been on holiday to Thailand.

123. A 26-year-old woman attends her GP. She has been encouraged to attend by her partner, although she suspects the lesion has been there life-long. There is a non-pigmented nodule at the lateral border of her eyebrow, which is being increasingly brought to her attention. It is not painful, and is smooth.

124. A 73-year-old woman, who spent much of her childhood in the sun attends her GP with a raised, pigmented nodule on her temple, the central core of which is darkest. It is firm but mobile, with regular edges.

Theme: Parotid pathology

A Adenocarcinoma of the parotid gland
B Frey's syndrome
C Lymphoma
D Pleomorphic adenoma of the parotid gland
E Sialoadenitis
F Sialolithiasis
G Sjögren's disease
H Sjögren's syndrome
I Warthin's tumour

Instructions: For each of the following scenarios, choose the single most likely diagnosis from the list above. Each option may be used once, more than once or not at all.

125. A 64-year-old man, who is a smoker, presents with a firm swelling of his left parotid. There is no apparent facial nerve weakness and the mass seems mobile overlying the sternomastoid muscle.

126. A 45-year-old woman with rheumatoid arthritis presents with a uniformly swollen right parotid gland. She is also reluctant to eat because of a dry mouth.

127. A 38-year-old man has previously undergone resection of a pleomorphic adenoma of his right salivary gland; he presents with recurrent swelling within the operative field, and also complains that when he eats, his face sweats on the right side.

Theme: Groin swellings

A Direct inguinal hernia
B Encysted hydrocele of cord
C Femoral hernia
D Hydrocele
E Incarcerated inguinal hernia
F Indirect inguinal hernia
G Inguinal lymphadenopathy
H Saphenovarix
I Varicocele

Instructions: For each of the following scenarios, choose the single most likely diagnosis from the list above. Each option may be used once, more than once or not at all.

128. A 74-year-old woman is admitted with a tender, non-reducible right groin swelling to the general surgical assessment unit. She has no symptoms of bowel obstruction.

129. A 2-year-old boy is seen by the paediatric surgeons. His mother is concerned that his scrotum appears intermittently swollen on the left, apparently worsened by a recent viral illness. The testicle remains palpable.

130. A 34-year-old man returns from foreign travel with a painful swollen right groin. There is a tender mass, which does not reduce, and which you can get 'above'. There is no cough impulse.

Theme: Gastrointestinal bleeding

A   Bleeding duodenal ulcer
B   Bleeding gastric ulcer
C   Boerhaave's syndrome
D   Crohn's disease
E   Distal colitis

F   Gastric carcinoma
G   Infective colitis
H   Ischaemic colitis
I   Mallory–Weiss tear
J   Oesophagitis

Instructions: For each of the following scenarios, choose the single most likely diagnosis from the list above. Each option may be used once, more than once or not at all.

131. A 28-year-old woman presents to the emergency department with a 2-week history of malaise, pyrexia and abdominal pain, and she now has increasing stool frequency with altered blood. She has a right iliac fossa mass.

132. An 80-year-old man presents acutely unwell with weight loss, lethargy, pain, but no abdominal tenderness, and melaena. He is a lifelong smoker. The abdominal X-ray is unremarkable but the stomach appears dilated.

133. A 22-year-old man, who has been binge drinking, and smokes, presents with a 2-day history of vomiting (with some blood noted).

Theme: Antimicrobial agents

A   Benzylpenicillin
B   Clindamycin
C   Flucloxacillin
D   Gentamicin
E   Meropenem

F   Metronidazole
G   None
H   Rifampicin
I   Tetracycline
J   Vancomycin

Instructions: For each of the following scenarios, choose the single most appropriate antibiotic from the list above. Each option may be used once, more than once or not at all.

134. A 64-year-old woman with minimal comorbidities presents with acute left iliac fossa peritonitis with localised signs only on the background of altered bowel habit. A CT diagnosis of locally contained, perforated sigmoid diverticulitis is made.

135. A 32-year-old man, known to be an intravenous drug abuser, is admitted to the medical assessment ward with tender, erythematous swelling, rapidly tracking from a groin injection site, and causing systemic sepsis.

136. A 67-year-old man needs to undergo upper gastrointestinal endoscopy to assess a likely hiatus hernia. He has a history of childhood rheumatic fever, and he had a porcine mitral valve replacement performed 8 years ago.

Theme: Risk assessment

A APACHE-II	**F** MODS
B ASA	**G** O-POSSUM
C CPEX	**H** P-POSSUM
D ISS	**I** RTS
E METS	**J** SAPS II

Instructions: For each of the following scenarios, choose the single most appropriate risk assessment scoring system from the list above. Each option may be used once, more than once or not at all.

137. A 43-year-old motorcyclist has been rescued by paramedics and has high-impact trauma. Based on his initial blood pressure, conscious level and respiratory rate, they bring him to a level 1 trauma centre.

138. A 72-year-old man has a potentially curable gastro-oesophageal cancer. He has severe osteoarthritis of the knees, but manages to mobilise reasonable distances. He would like to know his chance of surviving radical surgery.

139. A 58-year-old alcoholic woman has been in hospital for over a week, with worsening acute severe pancreatitis. She is transferred to the intensive care unit for ventilatory and renal support, whereas CT has demonstrated a necrotic pancreas. Her daughter recognises how ill her mother is, and wants to know her mother's chance of leaving hospital alive.

Theme: Nutrition

A   Elemental diet
B   Enteral feeding via fine bore
     nasogastric tube
C   Enteral feeding via fine bore
     nasogastric tube – overnight only
D   Enteral feeding via gastrostomy
E   Enteral feeding via surgically placed
     jejunostomy

F   Modular diet
G   Normal diet – no supplements
     required
H   Oral nutritional supplements
I   Total parenteral nutrition via
     Hickman/central line
J   Total parenteral nutrition via
     peripheral cannula

Instructions: For each of the following scenarios, choose the single most likely mode of nutrition from the list above. Each option may be used once, more than once or not at all.

140. A 54-year-old woman suffered from an acute severe episode of pancreatitis (85%) secondary to gallstones 2 months ago. This has resolved and she now tolerates oral diet without early satiety or vomiting. She has undergone successful laparoscopic cholecystectomy, but her nutritional state remains poor, with frequent diarrhoea and her body mass index is now 17 (reduced from 25).

141. A 36-year-old man has undergone multiple resections for Crohn's disease (most recently 3 months ago) and now presents with an enterocutaneous fistula, with minimal local abscess formation. Contrast studies define its course from midjejunum to skin, with an output of around 2 L of enteric content per day. His renal function is stable.

142. A 68-year-old man undergoes a potentially curative resection of a pancreatic head mass (by way of pylorus-preserving pancreaticoduodenectomy). He has a Malnutrition Universal Screening Tool (MUST) score of 2 preoperatively, and the operating team want to continue nutritional support in the early postoperative period.

Answers: SBAs

1. C Mesenteric ischaemia

Acute mesenteric ischaemia is a serious condition with a high morbidity and mortality. It can also be notoriously difficult to diagnose. CT of the abdomen with arterial contrast may show thickened loops of small bowel or thrombus in the involved arteries (coeliac axis, superior mesenteric artery or inferior mesenteric artery) (**Figure 1.1**).

A 10-year retrospective review of cases in the USA revealed 95% of cases presented with abdominal pain, and 44% had nausea. Vomiting and diarrhoea occurred in 35% of cases, tachycardia in 33%, and 16% had per rectal bleeding. Atrial fibrillation is strongly associated with mesenteric ischaemia as embolic cause accounts for 28% of cases and half of these patients are fibrillating.

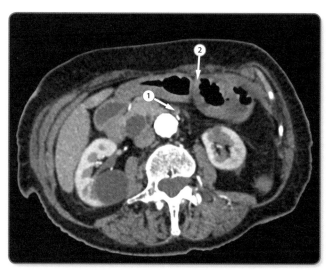

Figure 1.1 CT of small bowel ischaemia. ① Thrombus in superior mesenteric artery, ② Thickened small bowel.

2. A Age > 55 years

Age above 55 years alone is not predictive of the development of complications. Complications in acute pancreatitis occur more commonly in patients with clinical obesity. Complications are also more common in those patients with severe pancreatitis. This can be based on scoring systems (an APACHE II score > 8 in the first 24 hours after admission or a Glasgow Coma Score > 3). Severe pancreatitis also includes any organ failure which continues beyond 48 hours and a C-reactive protein > 150 mg/L. In both cases complications are more likely to occur.

3. C Defect in the pleuroperitoneal fold

A defect in the pleuroperitoneal fold may result in a posterolateral Bochdalek hernia which is the most common congenital diaphragmatic hernia, accounting for more than 95% of cases. The majority of Bochdalek hernias (78%) occur on the left side of the diaphragm, 20% on the right, and they are rarely bilateral. Unlike Morgagni herniae, Bochdalek herniae tend not to have a hernia sac. Morgagni herniae occur through the anterior space of Larrey.

4. A Calcium oxalate

Statistically, this stone is probably composed of calcium oxalate as this comprises 40% of ureteric calculi. Mixed oxalate/phosphate occurs in 20%, calcium phosphate and ammonium magnesium phosphate (struvite) stones both occur in 15% of patients and uric acid in 10%.

Stones containing calcium, such as calcium oxalate and calcium phosphate, are easiest to detect by radiography. Although 90% of urinary calculi have been considered to be radiopaque, the sensitivity and specificity of kidney, ureters, and bladder radiography alone remains poor (with sensitivity of 45–59% and specificity of 71–77%).

5. B Incidental mesenteric lesion found at laparoscopy/laparotomy

Meckel's diverticulae are normally 5 cm (2 inches) long pulsion diverticulae found approximately 60 cm (2 feet) from the ileocaecal valve on the antimesenteric border of the ileum. They occur in approximately 2% of the population and hence the 'Rule of 2s applies'. They represent an embryological remnant of the vitello-intestinal duct.

Most patients are asymptomatic although the Meckel's diverticulae can cause symptoms due to inflammation, bleeding or perforation. It can also present as the lead point for an intussusception or as the contents of an indirect inguinal hernia sac, in the eponymous Littre's hernia.

6. D Laparotomy

This patient has intestinal malrotation. This is a congenital condition occurring 1 in 500 live births, which can have serious complications. Malrotation occurs when there is a failure of embryological gut development and rotation, whereby the root of the mesentery remains narrow and the caecum occupies a non-rotated position in the right upper quadrant (**Figure 1.2**).

In the normal physiological state, starting from a straight tube, the embryological gut undergoes a complex series of rotations between 4–12 weeks culminating in the duodenojejunal flexure lying on the left side of the abdomen and the caecum positioned in the right iliac fossa.

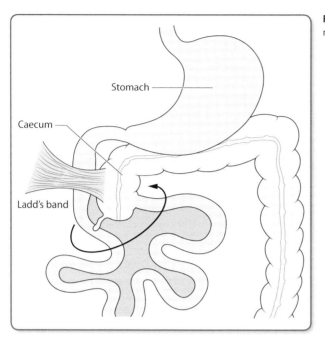

Figure 1.2 Intestinal malrotation.

There is a subsequent tendency for the bowel to twist around the mesentery and this combined with the development of adhesive Ladd's bands can lead to ischaemic bowel and perforation. As such early diagnosis is important to facilitate early laparotomy and avoid dangerous sequelae.

Operative repair involves division of the Ladd's band, appendicectomy, widening of the mesentery and relocation of the colon. A laparoscopic form of this procedure has evolved with the contrived acronym '**LADD**' (**L**aparoscopic **A**ppendicectomy and **D**uodenocolic **D**issociation).

7. C Excision with Roux-en-Y hepaticojejunostomy

Choledochal cysts are congenital dilations of the intra- and/or extrahepatic bile duct(s). They can be asymptomatic or present with components of the classic triad of jaundice, abdominal pain and right upper quadrant mass.

They can present in children or adults and have been classified by Todani et al. (1977) into types I–V (**Figure 1.3**):

- **Type I**: dilation of all or part of common bile duct (CBD; this is the most common form, representing 80–90% of all choledochal cysts).
- **Type II**: solitary cystic diverticulum extending from the CBD.
- **Type III**: arising from the duodenal CBD at its junction with the pancreatic duct.
- **Type IV**: cystic dilatations of the intra- and extrahepatic biliary tree.
- **Type V**: cystic dilatations of the intrahepatic biliary tree only.

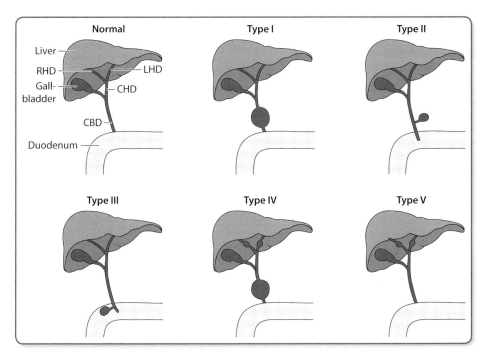

Figure 1.3 Choledochal cyst classification. RHD, right hepatic duct; LHD, left hepatic duct; CHD, common hepatic duct; CBD, common bile duct.

Children with choledochal cysts fare differently from adults as long-term complications are less common. The management of choledochal cysts used to involve internal drainage with cystoduodenostomy or cystoduodenotomy, but these procedures had a tendency to fail and up to 5% developed adenocarcinoma. The surgical treatment of choice is excision of the lesion and formation of a hepaticojejunostomy.

8. E Percutaneous drainage of abscess and intravenous antibiotics

In patients with an appendix mass there is a degree of clinical equipoise with regards to the specific management. The main treatment decisions are between:

- Immediate appendicectomy
- Conservative management with interval appendicectomy
- Conservative management alone.

The presence of an appendix abscess mandates either surgical or radiological drainage. In this patient's case there is a complex inflammatory mass and, as such, a surgical procedure would not be advisable.

9. E Trimethoprim

Trimethoprim is associated with hyperkalaemia. It inhibits the activity of the epithelial sodium channel resulting in elevated serum potassium. The four other drugs listed here as answer options are all associated with hypokalaemia rather than hyperkalaemia. Exposure to barium in the enema, antifungal treatment with amphotericin, diuretic therapy such as furosemide, and inhalers such as salbutamol, may all cause low potassium.

10. C Ongoing blood loss of 100 mL/min

Massive bleeding is defined as:

- Blood loss of half the patient's circulating volume in a 3-hour period
- Blood loss of the patient's circulating volume in a 24-hour period
- Ongoing blood loss of > 150 mL/min
- Transfusion of four units of packed red cells in a 4-hour period with continued bleeding
- Transfusion of 10 units of packed red cells in a 24-hour period.

A patient meeting such criteria should stimulate the activation of the local 'massive transfusion protocol'. This should alert the transfusion service to provide prompt delivery of packed red cells and suitable clotting products.

11. B Examination under anaesthesia and drainage of pus

Anorectal sepsis is a common presenting symptom which can present acutely as an abscess with erythema, pain and swelling or chronically as a fistula-in-ano. The peak incidence of perianal abscesses is in the third decade. Management of a perianal abscess is simple incision and drainage of underlying pus, whereas fistulotomy of a low fistula or insertion of a draining seton can be used if a fistula-in-ano is evident.

12. B A bladder pressure of 16–25 mmHg does not require decompression

As intra-abdominal pressure rises, so too does bladder pressure. Between 16 and 25 mmHg is grade 2 intra-abdominal hypertension, which normally manifests as oliguria. Recommended management at this stage includes fluid resuscitation, and if the pressure rises beyond the critical threshold of 25 mmHg, abdominal decompression is required (**Table 1.1**).

13. D Spontaneous detorsion of volvulus is common

Sigmoid volvulus has a characteristic inverted U-shape on plain abdominal X-ray (**Figure 1.4**). The management of sigmoid volvulus is relief of the obstruction, normally by sigmoidoscopic decompression. This technique is successful in 70–80% of cases. A rectal tube can be left in situ to reduce the chance of recurrence. Despite

Table 1.1 Abdominal compartment syndrome			
Grade	Bladder pressure (mmHg)	Clinical signs	Recommended management
I	<15	None	Maintain normovolaemia
II	16–25	Oliguria	Volume infusion
III	26–35	Anuria: ↓ cardiac output ↑ airway pressure	Decompression
IV	>35	Anuria: ↓ cardiac output ↑ airway pressure	Decompression/re-exploration

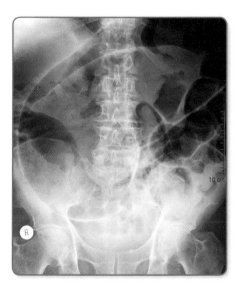

Figure 1.4 Sigmoid volvulus.

a successful result, volvulus recurs in 50–90% of patients, and as such this technique should be considered as a temporising measure only.

Following further medical assessment and resuscitation, a decision can be made to proceed to definitive surgery (removal of the sigmoid colon). This may also be indicated if the volvulus recurs, or cannot be decompressed.

Other therapeutic options include barium or water-soluble contrast enemas. This technique results in detorsion of the volvulus in approximately 5% of adults, although better results have been achieved in children. Spontaneous reductions in all patients are rare and occur in only 2% of patients.

14. B Extreme altitude

The oxygen haemoglobin dissociation curve represents the relationship between the partial pressure of oxygen and the oxygen saturation. The affinity of haemoglobin for oxygen increases as further molecules of oxygen are bound. This results in a sigmoid-shaped curve until no further oxygen can be bound.

When this curve is shifted to the left, this represents a higher affinity of haemoglobin for oxygen at that given pressure. Conversely, when this curve is shifted to the right this represents lower affinity and consequently oxygen is released to the tissues more readily.

The curve is shifted to the right by acidosis (decreased pH), increased temperature, increased 2,3-diphosphoglycerate and raised CO_2. This is analogous to exercising muscles and means that more oxygen is made available to the tissues. At extreme altitude the oxygen haemoglobin dissociation curve shifts to the left because there is much less CO_2 in the blood (**Figure 1.5**).

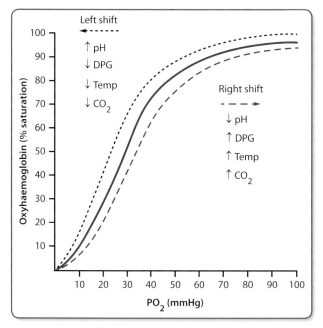

Figure 1.5 The oxygen haemoglobin dissociation curve. DPG; diphosphoglycerate.

15. A It contains clotting factors II, VII, VIII and IX

Prothrombin complex concentrate contains clotting factors II, VII, IX and X (the vitamin K-dependent factors). It also contains protein C and protein S. It is indicated for treatment, and perioperative prevention, of bleeding in patients with (acquired or congenital) deficiency of factors II, VII, IX or X, or if purified specific coagulation factors are not available.

16. D The immediate administration of adrenaline and noradrenaline will improve this patient's chance of survival

The administration of inotropes and vasopressors in a hypovolaemic patient causes myocardial hypoxia and cardiac dysfunction. Patients should have volume replacement once haemorrhage control is achieved. Inotropes may be required in cardiogenic shock when volume replacement is satisfactory.

The indications for resuscitative thoracotomy are penetrating injury to the chest or abdomen resulting in cardiac arrest, and blunt trauma leading to a peri-arrest/arrested low-flow state from haemorrhage uncontrollable by any other means.

Contraindications to resuscitative thoracotomy are a definite loss of cardiac output for >10 minutes, blunt trauma with no witnessed cardiac activity and severe head injury.

In patients undergoing resuscitative thoracotomy, isolated thoracic stab wounds causing cardiac tamponade have the highest survival rates (up to 70%). Gunshot wounds causing injury to more than one cardiac chamber have a higher mortality, as do injuries to the great vessels and pulmonary hila.

Patients in cardiac arrest will not require the induction of anaesthesia prior to intubation and ventilation. Those who are hypotensive but awake will require a rapid sequence induction of anaesthesia. The induction of anaesthesia may result in loss of blood pressure even when using ketamine or etomidate. Muscle relaxation is required throughout.

17. D CT of abdomen and pelvis

Diverticular disease is its complicated form can present with a patient showing clinical signs of sepsis and will require treatment with intravenous antibiotics. In severe sepsis combination antibiotics should be prescribed. In an unwell patient a CT of abdomen and pelvis can provide information as to the cause of the sepsis, i.e. confirming or refuting the suspected diagnosis as well as providing further details, such as any underlying abscesses which may be amenable to radiological drainage. A CT may also show any evidence of fistulation, obstruction or perforation, which may require more aggressive management.

18. E Subtotal colectomy and ileostomy

This patient has severe acute colitis and is systemically unwell. The treatment is an emergency subtotal colectomy and end ileostomy. She has failed medical management. Although there are a number of classifications for acute colitis, Truelove and Witts' classification (**Table 1.2**) provides a straightforward method of classification for such patients.

Table 1.2 Truelove and Witts' classification of severity of ulcerative colitis			
	Mild	Moderate	Severe
Bloody stools/day	<4	4–6	>6
Temperature	Apyrexial	Intermediate	>37.8°C
Heart rate	Normal	Intermediate	>90 bpm
Haemoglobin (g/L)	>110	105–110	<105
Erythrocyte sedimentation rate (mm/h)	<20	20–30	>30

19. D 13

The Glasgow Coma Scale is a 15-point scale for assessing and recording a patient's conscious state (**Table 1.3**). It is composed of eye opening, best motor and verbal response.

		Best motor response	Best verbal response	Eye opening
		Table 1.3 Glasgow Coma Scale		
		Best motor response	**Best verbal response**	**Eye opening**
6		Obeys commands	–	–
5		Localises painful stimuli	Orientated Normal conversation	–
4		Withdraws from painful stimuli	Confused Disorientated	Opens eyes spontaneously
3		Abnormal flexion to painful stimuli (decorticate response)	Inappropriate words	Responds to voice
2		Extends to painful stimuli (decerebrate response)	Incomprehensible sounds	Responds to pain
1		Makes no movements	No sounds	No eye opening

Adapted from: Teasdale G, Jennett B. Assessment of coma and impaired consciousness. A practical scale. Lancet 1974; 2: 81–84.

20. C Haemoglobin solution

Solutions of free haemoglobin do not have the antigenic characteristics of the blood groups, and they therefore do not require compatibility testing. ABO incompatibility can reduce the expected platelet count increment by 10–30%.

21. E Grade IV injury describes a laceration producing major devascularisation (> 25% of spleen)

Grade IV injury describes a laceration producing major devascularisation equivalent to over 25% of the spleen.

Grade I splenic injuries include subcapsular haematomas (of < 10% of the surface area) and capsular lacerations < 1 cm deep. Grade II splenic injuries include subcapsular haematomas (of < 50% of the surface area) and intraparenchymal haematomas < 5 cm. They also include capsular tears between 1 and 3 cm deep. Grade III splenic injuries include expanding subcapsular or intraparenchymal haematomas, ruptured haematomas, and any lacerations > 3 cm (or involving trabecular vessels). Grade IV injuries describe segmental, or hilar, vessel lacerations or major devascularisation. Grade V injuries refer to a completely shattered or devascularised spleen.

22. E Upper gastrointestinal endoscopy and proctoscopy

Acute colonic bleeding is a common problem and can manifest in a broad spectrum of clinical signs. The incidence increases with age and in the majority it resolves without intervention. However, in approximately 15% of cases bleeding will continue, resulting in haemodynamic instability. CT angiography has been shown in porcine models to detect bleeding rates of < 0.3 mL/min, but endoscopic visualisation of the upper gastrointestinal tract with endoscopy and proctoscopy should be first line investigations. Haemorrhoids must be excluded as a cause.

23. B Diverticular bleeding is the most common cause, accounting for approximately 50% of cases

In the elderly population the most common cause of massive colonic bleeding is diverticular disease, (up to 50% of cases) closely followed by angiodysplasia (40%) . The incidence of bleeding post polypectomy is < 2%.

24. E Signs of peritonitis suggest ischaemia or perforation

Large bowel obstruction is a common surgical emergency. Mechanical causes account for > 60%, colonic tumours account for 20% and volvulus 5%. Nausea and vomiting are late signs as the obstruction is distal in the gastrointestinal tract. CT has largely replaced other investigations as it can distinguish between different pathologies and, if the obstruction is the result of a malignant cause, it will provide information on staging.

25. B Colonic stenting

This is a frail patient with significant comorbidities, which would make any surgery very high risk. Even a loop colostomy is associated with significant morbidity and a small mortality rate. Stenting of the obstructing colonic lesion can achieve the same functional result as surgical decompression without the need for an operation and defunctioning colostomy. It can be used to allow time for work-up to definitive surgery or in an elderly patient, such as this, can provide good palliation.

26. B In low doses it increases renal blood flow

Dopamine has varying dose-related effects due to α_1-, β_1- and dopaminergic activity:

Low dose effects (at doses < 2 µg/kg/min) are predominantly renal. There is increased renal, cerebral, coronary and mesenteric blood flow with vasodilation because of agonistic action on dopamine receptors in these vascular beds.

Intermediate dose effects (at doses 2–10 µg/kg/min) are predominantly cardiac. β_1-agonist activity results in increased cardiac contractility and heart rate. The increased cardiac output and increased dopaminergic activity results in increased mesenteric perfusion. Slight α_1-adrenergic activity may lead to a degree of peripheral vasoconstriction.

High dose effects (at doses 10–20 µg/kg/min) are vasoconstrictive and cardiac. α_1-Adrenergic activity causes marked peripheral vasoconstriction and a rise in blood pressure. There can also be renal and mesenteric vasoconstriction. At very high doses (> 20 µg/kg/min) the overriding adrenergic activity may cause extreme vasoconstriction, which can suppress dopaminergic renal vasodilation and deleteriously affect the renal and peripheral circulation.

27. C In pT4 melanoma (> 4 mm thickness) an excision margin of 2 cm is recommended

For surgical excision of melanomatous lesions:

- In pTis (melanoma in situ) an excision margin of 2–5 mm is recommended
- In pT1 melanoma (0–1 mm thickness) an excision margin of 1 cm is recommended
- In pT2 melanoma (1–2 mm thickness) an excision margin of 1–2 cm is recommended
- In pT3 melanoma (2–4 mm thickness) an excision margin of 2 cm is recommended
- In pT4 melanoma (>4 mm thickness) an excision margin of 2 cm is recommended

In patients with squamous cell carcinoma, a 4 mm margin is sufficient to remove microscopic tumour in over 95% of well-differentiated tumours which are < 2 cm in diameter. A wider margin of 6–10 mm is required for lesions > 2 cm in diameter, less-differentiated, or in high-risk locations (such as the scalp, ears, eyelids, nose, or lips).

In cases of primary basal cell carcinoma (BCC), a 3 mm surgical margin adequately clears the tumour in 85% of patients with lesions <2 cm. However, increasing the excision margin to 4–5 mm increases the peripheral clearance rate to 95%.

In instances of recurrent BCC, margins of 5–10 mm have been recommended.

28. D Injection of cyanoacrylate glue

Unlike oesophageal varices, bleeding from gastric varices is difficult to treat using band ligation because of difficult deployment in a retroflexed scope position. There are few controlled studies of medical therapy for gastric variceal bleeding and most evidence is extrapolated from what is known regarding the management of oesophageal varices.

The best endoscopic therapy for fundal gastric variceal bleeding is injection of cyanoacrylate glue which hardens on contact with blood. Following healing, when the mucosa sloughs away the overlying glue 'cap' will also be shed. Complications include infection and embolism of glue particles (which are fortunately very rare). The glue can also harden inside the scope and this can damage the equipment.

29. D Retroperitoneal, between the ovarian vessels and the renal veins

Retroperitoneal varices occur between the mesenteric vessels and renal (or gonadal, or iliac) veins. However, in patients with infrarenal inferior vena cava obstruction, the ovarian (gonadal) vessels act as a collateral drainage for the systemic circulation by facilitating drainage form the internal iliac vessels to the left renal vein and the cava itself. However, this does not involve a portosystemic anastomosis.

Other sites of collateralisation (between the portal and systemic circulations) include:

- The rectum, where the superior rectal from inferior mesenteric vein anastomoses with the middle and inferior rectal veins/pudendal vein.
- The paraumbilical region, where the left portal/paraumbilical vein anastomoses with the vestigial umbilical vein/superficial epigastric and caput medusa may result.
- The distal oesophagus, where the left gastric vein anastomoses with oesophageal branches of the azygous vein.
- Intrahepatic, between the portal vein and the inferior vena cava.

30. A *Clostridium difficile*

Alcohol-based hand rubs are less effective on soiled hands and are ineffective against *Clostridium difficile* infection. The hand rub is unable to kill the bacterial spores.

31. A Addison's disease

This patient has biochemical evidence of metabolic acidosis with low bicarbonate, sodium and glucose and an elevated serum potassium. The normal range for serum glucose is 4–7 mmol/L.

Addison's disease (or adrenocortical insufficiency) results in reduced synthesis of mineralocorticoids and glucocorticoids. As a result of decreased glucocorticoid effects, there is a reduction in serum blood glucose. Because of decreased circulating cortisol, the kidney cannot excrete free water and hyponatraemia develops. Metabolic acidosis develops because of low aldosterone levels causing sodium loss in the urine, with H^+ retention in the serum. Low aldosterone also leads to hyperkalaemia. Clinical symptoms which develop are mainly due to the low blood sugar (hypoglycaemic autonomic effects) and low sodium (hypotension).

32. D Right hemicolectomy

The patient requires a right hemicolectomy as the carcinoid of the appendix is > 2 cm in diameter. A right hemicolectomy should be considered if the appendix tumour is large (1–2 cm) or invades the serosa. If a right hemicolectomy is to be performed then a regional lymphadenectomy should also be considered.

33. B Kruskall–Wallis test

When answering a statistical question, it is important to select the correct test (**Table 1.4**). In this example, a test for an association between two continuous variables is sought. Satisfaction scores (notoriously difficult to attain reliability) are very unlikely to have normal distribution, and so median scores are applicable. Therefore, without assuming equal variances or normal distribution in the data, the Kruskal–Wallis test can be applied; where normal distribution and mean values are applied, ANOVA would be the correct test. The Mann–Whitney U test compares medians in two sets of continuous data; the 2-sided t-test compares means and the linear regression analysis is applicable in determining the contribution of multiple factors to one continuous outcome variable.

Table 1.4 provides a simple overview for comparative statistical tests that should be easily remembered.

Table 1.4 Statistical tests for simple comparisons		
Comparison	**Measure**	**Test**
1 patient, 2 measures	Mean	Single sample t-test
1 patient, 2 measures	Median	Wilcoxon sign rank test
2 groups	Mean	Unpaired t-test
2 groups	Median	Mann–Whitney U test
2 proportions	%	χ^2
2 proportions – paired	%	McNemar test
>2 groups	Mean	ANOVA
>2 groups	Median	Kruskal–Wallis

34. A A significant difference (p-value = 0.05) has a likelihood of being due to chance in 1 in 20 cases

A type I (α) error describes the likelihood of wrongly rejecting the null hypothesis. A p-value of 0.05 describes the chance that a seemingly positive finding is actually due to luck alone, and in fact, no real difference exists (0.05 is equivalent to 1 in 20 mathematically).

It is clear that a power calculation has been carried out, based on the desired power and relevant difference which we wish to detect. The methodology described is that of a randomised controlled trial. In specially designed, pragmatic studies, either surgeon and/or patient preference may be accounted for, although this is not generally the case in controlled trials. Early stopping rules always apply, with patient safety being paramount. If there is clearly a higher rate of complication with the new intervention, a trial is not justified, as the whole basis for its carrying one out is that of clinical equipoise and uncertainty. If a trial is underpowered, there may be too few subjects to correctly identify a real difference. This is a false negative or falsely retaining the null hypothesis, and represents a type II (β) error.

35. A Case–control study

Here, we have a condition which we wish to link with a previous exposure. The question may be answered with a population level, longitudinal cohort study, following up children and recording details of any exposure, with rates of goitre later in life, to generate relative risk data. However, this is wholly impractical. It is more straightforward to answer this question by comparing two sets of odds ratios, to attribute the likelihood that someone with a condition has had a certain exposure, compared to the likelihood that someone free of the exposure has the condition. This does not imply causality, but degrees of relationship can be ascertained, and may provide justification for larger scale, longitudinal studies. Thus, the two sets of patients have different odds ratios generated. A randomised trial of exposure is simply unethical. An environmental study may act as a hypothesis-generating study during the early stages of studies. A meta-analysis may address the question, but would be unspecific to this surgeon's own population. It also traditionally pertains only to randomised controlled trials.

36. D Ensuring it represents a more general population

Although external validity describes the applicability of trial data to the broader population, it is widely acknowledged that participants in randomised controlled trials (RCTs) are not typical patients. These patients self-select (selection bias) as being more interested/motivated around their healthcare issues, and their treatment will be different, regardless of protocols. The Hawthorne effect describes the change in behaviour, and potential outcomes, experienced by both participants and clinicians involved in trials, by the very fact they are aware of being studied. The other options simply describe best practice to ensure internal validity in any RCT, and so all must apply for the results to be valid and reliable in themselves.

37. D Patients with prolonged hospital stays are at particular risk

Although vancomycin is rarely associated with *Clostridium difficile* diarrhoea, it is more often used as a second line treatment, after oral metronidazole. Prolonged hospital admissions (and in particular, stays in the intensive care unit), are independently associated *C. difficile* infection. The clinical presentation of this chapter ranges from mild diarrhoea, to severe pancolitis with pseudomembranes, sepsis and perforation. Examples of this are shown in the endoscopic (**Figure 1.6**) and postoperative (**Figure 1.7**) images. A low index of clinical suspicion is required for adequate infection control.

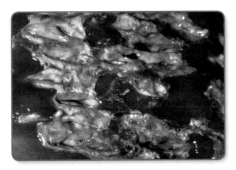

Figure 1.6 Endoscopic appearance of *Clostridium difficile* colitis. Pseudomembranes seen at colonoscopy, typical but not specific to *C. difficile* colitis.

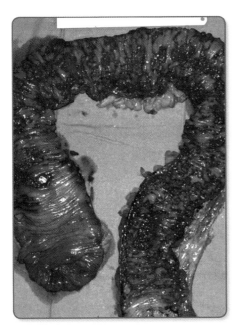

Figure 1.7 Resected colon with *Clostridium difficile* colitis. The end result of fulminant colitis, with a subtotal colectomy performed emergently.

38. B Formal diagnosis of malnutrition may be made with body mass index (BMI) ≤ 18 kg/m²

The NICE guideline CG32 (NICE; 2006) states that nutritional screening should be offered to all patients at the point of admission and if a clinical concern arises at any time, then subsequently repeated weekly for inpatients. A routine method to accomplish this is the Malnutrition Universal Screening Tool (MUST) (**Table 1.5**), based on the patient's body mass index (BMI), degree of unintentional weight loss, and effect of acute disease. This was developed to ensure a reliable, thorough and reproducible screening technique. Obese patients, as defined by BMI > 30, may still be malnourished in terms of loss of lean muscle mass, particularly in the acute illness phase. BMI ≤ 18 (or 20 with associated > 5% weight loss over 3–6 months), or weight loss > 10% in the same period are diagnostic. Patients require baseline trace elements to be checked only prior to commencement of parenteral feeding.

Step	Measure	Calculation
	Table 1.5 Calculation of the MUST score	
1	Body mass index	BMI > 20 = 0 18.5–20 = 1 < 18.5 = 2
2	Weight loss (unplanned weight loss in the past 3–6 months)	% weight loss: < 5 = 0 5–10 = 1 > 10 = 2
3	Acute illness (if patient is acutely ill and there has been no nutritional intake for >5 days)	= 2
4	Overall risk of malnutrition	Add scores from steps 1–3 to calculate the overall risk of malnutrition

Score 0, low risk; score 1, medium risk; score 2 or more, high risk. Adapted from: Malnutrition Advisory Group. Malnutrition Universal Screen Tool. Redditch, Worcestershire: British Association for Parenteral and Enteral Nutrition; 2003.

39. D Prevalence: risk of developing a new condition within a specified period

This describes incidence, not prevalence. Odds ratios and relative risks are frequently confused. Odds ratios pertain to retrospective data, working back from an event to assess the likelihood of having been exposed to a risk factor. They cannot be used to describe aetiology with certainty, and are useful in hypothesis generation and epidemiological studies. Relative risk ratios are calculated over prospective, longitudinal data, and reliably inform the strength of the relationship between exposure and outcomes. The absolute risk reduction is a numerical calculation, subtracting the risk rate in the control group from that in a study group. This may then be used to calculate the number needed to treat, which indicates the number of patients who require exposure to an intervention in order for any one patient to benefit. This is useful in economic modelling. Straus et al. (2010) provides a readable guide to putting these numbers into practice.

40. C. Hyaluronidase

Extravasation is a common occurrence in hospitals, potentially affecting up to 39% of inpatients. However, most cases do not require treatment other than stopping the infusion and removing the cannula. The degree of cellular injury depends on the volume and type of solution being infused. TPN is a hyperosmolar agent. Extravasation is treated with hyaluronidase 15 units/mL as 0.2 mL subcutaneous injection near the extravasation site

41. A Pa_{CO_2} of > 7 kPa has been documented

The Pa_{CO_2} need rise only to 6–6.5 kPa to confirm brainstem death. The other criteria are accurate. In the UK, brainstem death is defined as complete, irreversible loss of brainstem function, made according to well-defined criteria and preconditions, with reversible causes of apnoeic coma excluded, and brainstem areflexia and persistent apnoea confirmed. The cranial nerve reflexes tested are set out in **Table 1.6**.

Table 1.6 Cranial nerve testing in brainstem death		
Reflex	**Test**	**Nerves**
Pupillary	Direct and consensual response to light	II III
Corneal	Blink stimulation with cotton wool	V, VII
Vestibulo-ocular	Otoscopy to confirm to obstruction, then, instillation of ice-cold water to external auditory canals with eyelids held open – no eye movement	III, VI, VIII
Supraorbital grimace	No grimacing or motor response with firm supraorbital pressure	V VII (Peripheral stimuli may result in an apparent response, which is a spinal reflex – this does not preclude diagnosing brainstem death)
Gag/cough reflex	Deep tracheal suction via endotracheal tube	IX/X

42. B Obese patients (BMI > 30) should be excluded from day case lists

Obese patients were originally excluded from day case surgery lists, with BMI limits varying considerably between units. A BMI of 30–40 was used as a cut-off, but increasingly even super-obese patients are being managed as day cases. It is now deemed acceptable to make this judgement on an individual patient basis. The other statements correctly describe defined criteria. Full details are available from the anaesthetic guidelines (Verma et al., 2011) for day case surgery.

43. A The caecum fails to descend to a subhepatic position during embryological development

Malrotation (Figure 1.2), although commonly presenting in the first few months of life, may also present at a later stage, with 0.2% presenting much later in adulthood. When it presents in the neonatal period and the first few months of life, it constitutes a surgical emergency, and although baseline evaluation of biochemical and haematological indices are recommended, they should not delay surgery. Radiological investigations typically show a gasless abdomen, with a little stomach gas an isolated feature; contrast studies make the definitive diagnosis, normally demonstrating a 'corkscrew' duodenum with the duodenojejunal flexure lying to the right of the midline. It is usually an isolated abnormality and the child will go on lead a normal life following surgical correction.

44. E It most commonly occurs in an ileocolic segment of bowel

The most common cause of paediatric intussusception is lymphoid hyperplasia in the Peyer's patches of the gut. The most prominent such tissue occurs along the ileocaecal segment (**Figure 1.8**). Hence, this is not a congenital 'lead point' for the intussusception as such. Other possible lead points include Meckel's diverticulum and duplication cysts, as well as B lymphoma of the gut. Intussusception most commonly presents in the 2 months to 2 years age bracket. A high level of diagnostic accuracy is achieved with abdominal ultrasound, which may demonstrate the 'target' sign of bowel within bowel.

Pneumatic reduction ('air enema') is routinely attempted unless the child already has signs of perforation or peritonitis, in which case operative reduction is necessary. Prior to pneumatic reduction, intravenous access should be secured and the patient prepared for theatre in case it becomes necessary to resort to an operative approach. Often operative reduction is achieved without any need to resect bowel.

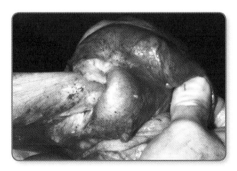

Figure 1.8 Intussusception. Characteristic ileocolic intussusception necessitating operative reduction with or without resection following assessment of bowel viability.

45. C Laparotomy in emergency theatre

This patient requires an urgent laparotomy [the Advanced Trauma Life Support manual (American College of Surgeons; 1997)]. He is haemodynamically unstable, with evidence of fluid loss (probably blood) and peritonitis, indicating significant intra-abdominal injury. Scans will delay definitive management and may be dangerous in this context. No useful information will be gleaned from a FAST scan to supplement the clear clinical signs. Delayed pancreatitis is associated with blunt trauma to the same region. Catheterisation will take place perioperatively, irrespective of the pathology.

46. E The blood supply of a Meckel's diverticulum is from the omphalomesenteric artery

Meckel's diverticulum is the most common congenital abnormality, present in 2% of the population and is located 60 cm proximal to the ileocaecal valve. It is caused by the incomplete obliteration of the vitelline duct. The vitelline duct should close by 7 weeks' gestation. A Meckel's diverticulum may contain ectopic mucosal tissue. It may cause gastrointestinal bleeding (in younger children), or inflammation, obstruction, intussusception or even perforation. In older children, the presentation may mimic appendicitis.

A technetium-99m (Tc-99m) pertechnetate scintiscan is used for diagnostic purposes. Pertechnetate is taken up by heterotopic gastric mucosa if the diverticulum contains this ectopic tissue. Accuracy of the scan may be enhanced with administration of cimetidine which enhances the uptake and blocks the secretion of Tc-99m pertechnetate from ectopic gastric mucosa.

The blood supply of a Meckel's diverticulum is from the omphalomesenteric artery, a remnant of the vitelline artery which originates from the ileal branch of the superior mesenteric artery.

47. C Infants present with a hypochloraemic, hypokalaemic metabolic alkalosis

Infantile hypertrophic pyloric stenosis is a common surgical problem, and often managed by the non-specialist paediatric general surgeon by way of Ramstedt's pyloromyotomy (**Figure 1.9**). The precise aetiology remains unknown, but it tends to affect first-born males, some with a family history, at around 4–6 weeks of age. The vomiting is specifically non-bilious in nature. The child usually has been thriving, until insidious onset of vomiting, which then becomes projectile. The speed of presentation for medical help often determines the degree of metabolic disturbance, but the prolonged loss of gastric juices leads to an alkalosis, with potassium also lost in exchange for the kidney's attempt to preserve chloride. Electrolyte correction, specifically of the hypochloraemia, and volume replacement must be carried out prior to surgical intervention, which may be delayed by a number of days if necessary. Recovery following the pyloromyotomy is normally straightforward.

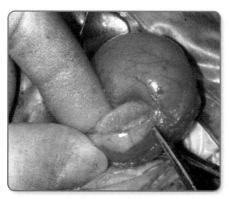

Figure 1.9 Ramstedt's pyloromyotomy, demonstrating the incision through the serosa, down to the pouting mucosa, overlying the hypertrophic pyloric segment.

48. A A child with peritonitis should have volume resuscitation (≥ 20 mL/kg intravenous fluid) prior to surgery

This describes the correct fluid resuscitation of any acutely unwell child. Prior to anaesthesia (in the context of sepsis/peritonitis) some volume resuscitation is always required. There is no absolute age below which a laparoscopic approach is contraindicated, but its use must depend on the expertise of the surgeon, with the small abdominal cavity and stretchy parietal peritoneum posing specific considerations.

Despite there being fewer differential diagnoses in the paediatric presentation of appendicitis, the behaviour of the disease is different. This is especially true in the very young, and often presents at a more advanced stage (**Figure 1.10**). This perhaps in part reflects difficulties in communication causing a delay in reaching a diagnosis. Active observation, formally reported over 30 years ago, remains the most important diagnostic tool. There is no substitute for repeated reassessment of subjective and objective signs. No one serological or radiological test is entirely reliable.

As in adults, presentation with advanced disease is not uncommon in the paediatric population, and laparoscopic appendicectomy can be safely performed in the majority of such cases.

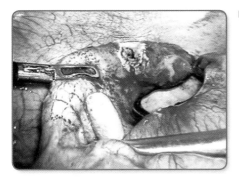

Figure 1.10 Paediatric appendicitis.

49. D Medial visceral rotation manoeuvres may be required to fully inspect the retroperitoneum

The principles of damage control surgery are to control haemorrhage, prevent contamination and avoid further injury. Patients should undergo operative management quickly without unnecessary delays for imaging or attempts at resuscitation. Only investigations that will immediately influence management should be undertaken.

They should be prepped and draped from neck to knees, and only then should anaesthesia be induced. Immediate four quadrant packing may be required to control haemorrhage, as may aortic control, best achieved at the diaphragmatic hiatus.

Careful inspection of the abdominal cavity is mandatory and may require medial visceral rotations to fully facilitate this. Nonexpanding perirenal haematomas, retrohepatic haematomas or blunt pelvic haematomas should not be explored and may be treated with abdominal packing. Angiographic embolisation may be required.

Contamination should be managed with simple suture or stapled resection of damaged bowel. Anastomoses should not be undertaken.

Abdominal closure should be rapid and temporary as re-look laparotomy is likely to be required. If there is concern over intra-abdominal compartment syndrome a laparostomy should be formed.

50. D Log roll including checking spinal integrity and anal tone

Within the Advance Trauma Life Support (ATLS) protocol (American College of Surgeons, 1997), primary survey, and any immediate resuscitative measures work in parallel, and only once each of the five components of the primary survey are 'stabilised' may the trauma provider move on to the more detailed secondary survey.

Primary survey includes:

- Airway assessment and maintenance with C-spine control
- Breathing assessment and ventilation if required
  - This includes assessment of respiratory rate and symmetry, with inspection, percussion and auscultation of the lung fields
- Circulation with haemorrhage control
  - This is assessed via conscious level, skin color and pulse, with external haemorrhage identified and controlled
- Disability: rapid assessment of neurological status
  - This is assessed via **AVPU** (**A**lert /responds to **V**oice /responds to **P**ain / **U**nresponsive) and pupillary responses
- Exposure/environmental control
- Full exposure of the patient, with re-warming as necessary

ABCDE describes the order of priority, and, if a prior element deteriorates, the algorithm is repeated in order as required. Secondary survey is only instigated once the patient is stabilised and resuscitation is in progress – allowing more time for a detailed, systematic evaluation, of which the log roll and associated check is part. A focused assessment with sonography for trauma (FAST) scan of the abdomen is an adjunct to the secondary survey, but increasingly being replaced by CT.

51. D Airway management – prepare for definitive orotracheal airway and have surgical airway kit ready

This patient has an emergency need for definitive airway control. He is alert to painful stimuli and therefore he is unsuitable for a Guedel airway. A nasopharyngeal airway is relatively contraindicated given the pattern of injuries (as would be a nasotracheal airway). If his airway is compromised by trauma, then a surgical airway may still be required, but a definitive orotracheal route is preferable with expertise available from anaesthetics. Until the airway is secured, there is little point in enhancing ventilation, and this is a secondary priority. However, until the airway is secured, every effort should be made to enhance oxygen delivery, and this may be carried out if enough personnel are available. It is not, however, the chief priority.

52. E Written consent must be taken prior to commencing CPEX

Cardiopulmonary exercise testing (CPEX) is used to establish exercise limitation, establish the underlying causes of respiratory compromise, and monitor functional status in cardiovascular disease. The patient is attached to an ECG, a facemask connected to a gas analyser, a pulse oximeter and a sphygmomanometer. Incremental exercise testing is performed on a treadmill or cycle ergometer. CPEX provides measurements of oxygen (O_2) consumption, carbon dioxide (CO_2) production, and lung ventilation. Absolute contraindications include myocardial infarction within the previous 5 days, acute myocarditis, severe symptomatic aortic stenosis, uncontrolled heart failure/arrhythmia, dissection aneurysm or resting oxygen saturations <86%. Patients should avoid food, nicotine and caffeine for 2 hours prior to testing.

VO_2 at anaerobic threshold of >11 mL/kg/min is a predictor of low cardiovascular risk after major abdominal surgery.

Risk of death during CPEX is 1:10000 and risk of acute myocardial infarction is 1:2500, therefore written consent must be obtained prior to testing.

53. D Noradrenaline is frequently the agent of choice in septic shock

Noradrenaline is the most commonly used inotrope in sepsis with hypoperfusion, predominantly acting at α-adrenoceptors to produce vasoconstriction to counter the hypotension that results from peripheral vasodilatation. The description in (B) applies to dobutamine, which is used in cardiac failure to reduce afterload. Adrenaline stimulates both α- and β-receptors, with respective vasoconstriction and enhanced cardiac contractility. Afterload may be increased, along with myocardial oxygen demands, so that it is not a useful agent in cardiogenic shock. Glyceryl trinitrate is a useful agent in cardiac failure, but through increased availability of nitric oxide, preload is reduced due to vasodilatation and reduced venous return. Dopexamine, active at $β_2$-receptors, aids in splanchnic perfusion, often in the context of cardiac failure. A concise summary of inotropic agents is given in Ashford and Evans (2001).

54. D Hyperthermia

Massive transfusion is associated with the 'lethal triad' of hypothermia, coagulopathy and metabolic acidosis. This is classically described in the rapid deterioration of severely injured patients, leading to a significant mortality rate when present.

Massive transfusion occurs when half of a patient's circulating volume is transfused in a period <24 hours. There is a requirement for close monitoring and optimisation of volume status and tissue oxygenation, as well as control of any bleeding or coagulation abnormalities. There may also be altered levels of ionised calcium or potassium, and the acid–base balance may be affected. There is a tendency for hyperkalaemia, hypokalcaemia and hypomagnesaemia (in part due to the citrate infused).

55. A A heart rate of >90 beats per minute and respiratory rate of >20 breaths per minute are adequate diagnostic criteria for SIRS

Although the definition of systemic inflammatory response syndrome (SIRS) is somewhat arbitrary, it represents the beginning of a potentially important continuum which may result in multiorgan failure if the process is not abated. SIRS is defined by the presence of two or more of the factors listed in **Table 1.7**. It was a working definition designed to help the early diagnosis of critically ill patients, derived from a consensus conference of physicians and intensivists in the USA 25 years ago (ACCP and SCCM, 1992).

SIRS is driven by the release and effect of inflammatory mediators such as interleukin-1 and 6, prostaglandins and leukotrienes, as well as catecholamines and insulin. Sepsis is the equivalent clinical state in the presence of bacteraemia. SIRS may occur in response to any systemic insult, such as major surgery, pancreatitis, trauma, etc. Organ dysfunction is frequently evident, but multiorgan dysfunction syndrome, and eventual multiorgan failure can result. Disseminated intravascular coagulation represents a failing haematological system and would not necessarily be seen in SIRS. Vasodilatation is characteristic, with nitric oxide mediated effects.

Table 1.7 Criteria for diagnosis of systemic inflammatory response syndrome	
Parameter	**Range required to define SIRS**
Core temperature	$<36°C$ or $>38°C$
Heart rate	>90 beats per minute
Ventillation	Respiratory rate >20 breaths per minute, or $Paco_2 < 4.26$ kPa
White cell count	$>12 \times 10^9$/L or $<4 \times 10^9$/L, with $>10\%$ immature forms

56. D Reduced blood pressure and cardiac output is an important side effect

Reduced blood pressure and cardiac output is an important side effect of positive pressure ventilation. Increased preload with reduced venous return occurs because of the loss of negative pressure in the intrathoracic pump.

Owing to reduced cardiac output, there is reduced renal blood flow, with reduced perfusion, urine output, and potential worsening of any acute injury in the context of acute illness. Although $Paco_2$ may arbitrarily be considered a reasonable threshold for consideration of ventilatory support, the decision to ventilate a patient is individual, and in the context of obstructive airways disease, this may be either non-critical, or relatively contraindicative, of support. Patients with injuries with raised intracranial pressure may be ventilated at low pressure and high frequency, to drive a reduction in CO_2 which will then reduce cerebral blood volume, and consequently pressure. Through ventilation alone, intrathoracic pressure increase will lead to increased intracranial pressures. Through more rapid correction of hypoxia, hypercapnia and acidosis, ventilation decreases the endogenous catecholamine drive on the cardiovascular system. This subsequently reduces the impact of the body's own stress response.

57. A Flail chest is defined radiographically as three or more consecutive ribs fractured in two or more places

Flail chest is defined radiographically as three or more consecutive ribs fractured in two or more places.

Rib fractures usually occur in association with pulmonary contusions, haemothorax, pneumothorax and blunt cardiac injury. The most common is pulmonary contusions.

Open reduction and internal fixation of rib fractures should be considered in those with five or more rib fractures and a flail, especially in patients requiring noninvasive or invasive positive pressure ventilation. Other indications include inadequate pain management associated with respiratory compromise, symptomatic nonunion, and thoracotomy for another pathology.

Patients with flail chest may require to be treated with either noninvasive or invasive positive pressure ventilation. They do not always require intubation.

58. B 4.5 L compound crystalloid over 8 hours, and the same again over the next 16 hours

This patient has sustained 27% body surface, partial thickness burns (**Figure 1.11**). This is a significant volume burn (despite his apparent stability) and he is at risk of delayed metabolic sequelae. The goal of management is continued urine production around 1 mL/kg/h for the first day and to monitor this all patients require urinary catheters. The Parkland formula is used by the ATLS protocol (see answer 50), whereby % burn × kg weight × 4 = minimum volume to be infused in first 24 hours postburn. The first half of this volume should be given in the first 8 hours and the second half in the next 16 hours. If the patient appears volume deplete at the outset, these proportions may be varied, and may be titrated against urinary output.

In this patient's case, he requires: 27% × 80 kg × 4 = 8640 mL total fluid

This equates to 4.32 L in first 8 hours, and the same in the subsequent 16 hours.

The simple charts in **Figure 1.11** provide an easy estimate for the % burn sustained – the higher surface area: volume ratio of children is important.

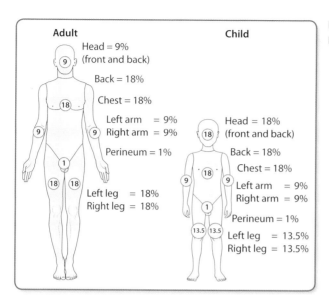

Figure 1.11 Calculating percentage burns.

59. E Night-time discharge from the intensive care unit is associated with poorer patient outcomes

Intensive care units provide level 3 care. Level 1 care is ward based and level 2 is high dependency care. Intensive care units should have a consultant to patient ratio less than 1:14. A lower ratio than this is detrimental to both patient care and consultant well being.

Following the decision for admission to the intensive care unit, admission should happen within 4 hours. Not all units will provide extracorporeal membrane oxygenation (ECMO). This is used to support cardiac and pulmonary failure.

Night-time discharge is associated with poorer patient outcomes and ideally patients should not be discharged from the intensive care unit between 22:00 and 07:00.

60. C Placement of a caval filter prior to return to theatre for anastomotic leak

This man has systemic compromise from his anastomotic leak. This will not settle with conservative management, and he therefore needs to return to theatre for control of sepsis and defunctioning. To do this safely, in the presence of a venous thrombosis, further prophylaxis against embolism is required. Emergency placement of a caval filter is also required. Low-molecular-weight heparin cannot be reversed, but this should neither preclude surgical intervention for his sepsis, nor filter placement. The evidence for filters is relatively weak but is outlined in Young et al. (2010).

61. A Abdominal compartment syndrome

The inflammatory response and intra-abdominal swelling which occurs secondary to acute severe pancreatitis is driving the pathophysiology in this scenario. Abdominal compartment pressure may be estimated by elevation of a urinary catheter from the level of the pubis. A pressure above 12 cm is elevated and > 20 cm is diagnostic of abdominal compartment syndrome (ACS). By reducing abdominal blood flow and diaphragmatic movement, the secondary compromise in renal and respiratory function are worsened, and pose particular management problems in terms of ventilating the patient against this increased pressure. The renal impairment remains acute, but is more complex than a straightforward acute renal injury. The form of pancreatitis is immaterial to the pathological outcome here. This phenomenon is increasingly recognised, and actively managed, in the acute surgical patient, often using a vacuum-assisted closure device (**Figure 1.12**). This image shows a typical sealed management system for management of the abdomen in a trauma patient for whom primary closure would be too dangerous.

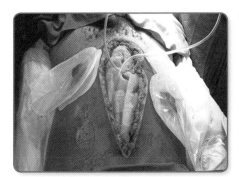

Figure 1.12 Management of an open abdomen.

Answers: EMIs

62. A Adhesions

The history of Crohn's disease is slightly misleading as there are no features here to suggest a 'flare-up' or recurrent disease. A more protracted history of pain or discomfort with increased bowel frequency and blood or mucus in the motions would be more classical and suggestive of active disease. Here the relevant history is of multiple laparotomies which will predispose the patient to the development of adhesions. Similar questions may push the candidate for a suitable management plan in the above clinical scenario. Most texts agree on a period (normally < 24 hours) of conservative management, including resting of the gastrointestinal tract, fluid resuscitation (with or without nasogastric aspiration or drainage if large volume or repeated vomits feature).

63. F Gallstone ileus

In patients aged over 65 years, gallstone ileus makes up approximately 25% of non-strangulated small bowel obstruction and carries a high mortality rate (approximately 15%). The unusual gas pattern seen here probably refers to pneumobilia (or gas in the biliary tree), and the opacification in the right lower quadrant is likely to represent a gallstone lodged in the terminal ileum. In conjunction with dilated fluid-filled loops of small bowel, these are classical radiographic findings associated with gallstone ileus. Despite this, the sensitivity of a plain radiograph for diagnosis of gallstone ileus varies from 40–70%. This compares to CT, which has a sensitivity and diagnostic accuracy of close to 100%.

64. J Pseudomyxoma peritonei

Pseudomyxoma peritonei (PMP) is a rare clinical entity affecting approximately one individual per million population. It is a form of malignancy characterised by mucin production which can progress to fill the abdomen and compress hollow organs. When picked up intraoperatively, the findings are surprising as the volume of mucinous material can be quite marked. Some people develop symptoms as a result of direct compression but PMP is considered only borderline malignant due to its slow clinical progression. It is associated with appendiceal and mucinous ovarian tumours and should always be suspected in patients with these diagnoses. Treatment is usually based on minimising symptoms and 'watchful waiting', unless progression is marked or the symptoms dictate intervention. In such cases, the Sugarbaker procedure (peritonectomy) is used for debulking with postoperative chemotherapy (often intraperitoneally).

65. B χ^2 test

When addressing a research question, it is important to differentiate between 'parametric' and 'non-parametric' data before selecting the appropriate method of description and the most accurate statistical test (**Table 1.8**). 'Parametric' refers

Table 1.8 Choosing a statistical test			
	Parametric measure/ test	**Non-parametric measure/test**	**Binomial measure/test**
Description of data location/distribution in one group	Mean/standard deviation	Median/interquartile range	Fraction/proportion
Comparison of 2 unpaired groups	Unpaired *t*-test	Mann–Whitney	Fisher's/χ^2
Comparison of 2 paired groups	Paired *t*-test	Wilcoxon	McNemar's
Comparison of ≥3 unmatched groups	One-way ANOVA	Kruskal–Wallis	χ^2
Comparison of ≥3 matched groups	Repeat-measures ANOVA	Friedman	–
Evaluate the association between 2 variables	Pearson correlation	Spearman rank correlation	–

to data which is normally distributed and follows Gaussian distribution, unlike 'non-parametric' data which is positively or negatively skewed. For practical purposes this can be determined by visualising the distribution of data on a histogram using a statistical package.

Parametric tests of normally distributed data include (Student's) paired *t*-test and independent *t*-test, which assess the distribution and central location of data between paired and unpaired cases respectively.

χ^2 testing is a comparison of proportions and is independent of whether data is normally distributed or not. However, it is restricted in its accuracy when values are low, and in such cases a Fisher's exact test must be used.

66. G Mann–Whitney U test

The Mann–Whitney U test is a non-parametric statistical test used to assess whether two independent samples of observations have differing values. Contrast this with the Wilcoxon signed-rank test, which is a non-parametric statistical test for two related samples or repeat observations on a single sample.

67. C Friedman's test

Friedman's test is a non-parametric test also used to detect differences between several related samples, or in one sample across repeated time points.

68. B Abdominal ultrasound

Following laparoscopic cholecystectomy, complications are relatively common and imaging studies may be required to assess for the presence of a fluid collection (which may represent abscesses, bilomas, or haematomas). These will not always require intervention as a small collection is commonly seen in the postoperative period. The easiest way to assess non-invasively is through abdominal ultrasound, which will provide information on the presence and amount of any collection and can also describe its homogeneity. As a first line investigation it is also useful for identifying a retained stone or any biliary dilation.

69. H CT of the abdomen

Although this patient has had a recent hernia operation, the medical history of diverticular disease cannot be ignored, particularly in view of the tenderness. A CT of the abdomen with intravenous and oral contrast should be performed to reject or confirm a diagnosis of diverticulitis. Pericolic fat infiltration is a diagnostic feature. Chronic pain following hernia repair does not tend to occur as high as the iliac fossa or lower quadrant, unless there is large or small bowel involvement.

70. H CT of the abdomen

If an anastomotic leak (and possible collection or abscess) is suspected, a CT of the abdomen and pelvis with intravenous, oral, and rectal contrast is indicated. This is a highly sensitive (95%) test for identifying abdominal or pelvic abscesses. It also affords the opportunity for CT-guided drainage, which is successful in up to 85% of patients.

Gastrografin enema is another commonly used technique which will provide information on the presence of a leak, but will not demonstrate if there is a drainable collection and further imaging will be required. This patient has evidence of sepsis and the tenderness suggests there may be a collection or abscess. This will require drainage and, depending on the extent of the leak, and the integrity of the anastomosis, a laparotomy for drainage or defunctioning may be required.

71. A Amyand's

Amyand is reported to have performed the first appendicectomy in 1735, on a patient with a perforated appendix situated in an inguinal hernia. This condition is very rare with an appendix in the sac of an inguinal hernia reported in approximately 1% of patients when the appendix is non-inflamed (and 0.08% when inflamed).

72. G Maydl's

A Maydl's hernia occurs when a 'W-shaped' segment of small bowel occupies the hernia sac. The middle part is situated inside the abdomen and may become strangulated, as can also happen to the adjacent loops of small bowel (**Figure 1.13**).

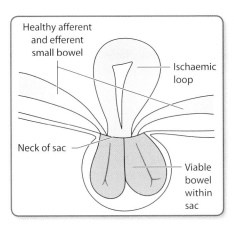

Figure 1.13 Maydl's hernia.

Labels in figure:
- Healthy afferent and efferent small bowel
- Ischaemic loop
- Neck of sac
- Viable bowel within sac

73. H Pantaloon

A Pantaloon hernia is a combination of direct and indirect herniae. The hernial sacs bulge on either side of the inferior epigastric vessels like 'pantaloons'.

74. H Hepatitis B surface antigen

Hepatitis B surface antigen (HBsAg) is a baseline diagnostic test to differentiate between ongoing or resolved hepatitis B in unwell patients. This test is used to determine the transmissibility of hepatitis B.

75. G Hepatitis B surface antibody

Hepatitis B surface antibody (anti-HBsAg) is a test to assess response to immunisation in healthcare workers. Such 'at-risk' groups of people receive three vaccinations of the hepatitis B surface antigen (HBsAg) at 1 and 6 months intervals. The hepatitis B surface antibody usually becomes measurable in the serum about 4 weeks after HBsAg is no longer measurable.

When antibody is present, it suggests that the infection is no longer active and the subject is immune to hepatitis B infection. It is therefore used to determine the need for further vaccination.

76. A Hepatitis C virus (HVC) polymerase chain reaction (PCR)

HCV PCR is a test used by hepatologists and virologists to monitor hepatitis C treatment by measuring the expression of HCV RNA.

77. J Magnetic resonance cholangiopancreatography (MRCP)

This patient has recurrent upper abdominal pain, with a recent ultrasound showing stones in the gallbladder. She is apyrexial with normal inflammatory markers and is therefore unlikely to have cholecystitis or cholangitis. With grossly abnormal liver function test values, she is likely to have ductal stones. There seems little value in repeating an ultrasound scan as the only difference to management would be if it clearly demonstrated ductal stones with dilatation requiring decompression.

MRCP utilises magnetic resonance imaging to examine the biliary and pancreatic tree in great detail, although it does not offer any therapeutic options. Compared to an invasive procedure like ERCP, there is very minimal mortality or morbidity with MRCP. Performing this procedure will provide information on the presence of any ductal stones and will therefore guide the need for further treatment. A major limiting factor in patients undergoing MRCP is that some will require a subsequent ERCP regardless.

78. D ERCP with balloon trawl with or without sphincterotomy

This woman presents with acute cholecystitis and a dilated common bite duct (CBD) (based on her ultrasound findings). She will require a cholecystectomy at some point, but her biliary tree needs decompressed and this should be performed with endoscopic retrograde cholangiopancreatography (ERCP) (**Figure 1.14**).

This patient is high risk as her CBD is dilated beyond 10 mm. As with other high-risk patients (with cholangitis or pancreatitis) she should undergo ERCP +/− duct decompression. Up to a third of such patients will have no evidence of a gallstone at ERCP and further tests may be required at a later date.

79. G Laparoscopic cholecystectomy with on-table cholangiogram

This patient is at low risk of gallstone-related complications and should proceed to cholecystectomy without further preoperative diagnostic procedures. He should also have an intraoperative cholangiogram (IOC) to demonstrate any distal common bite duct (CBD) or pancreatic duct stones.

80. H Pilonidal sinus

Pilonidal disease can be asymptomatic, or may present with an abscess or discharging sinus tract (most commonly in the natal cleft region). It occurs due to ingrowing hairs and is more common in male, hirsute patients who sit for prolonged periods.

81. B Anal fissure

An anal fissure is a small tear or ulcer at the anal verge (normally in the 6 o'clock position). It has been suggested it is due to ischaemia with impaired healing due to a combination of increased sphincter tone, fibrotic scarring and repeated mechanical injury. When an anal fissure develops, it may cause severe sharp pain on defaecation which can last for hours afterwards. There may also be fresh blood on the toilet

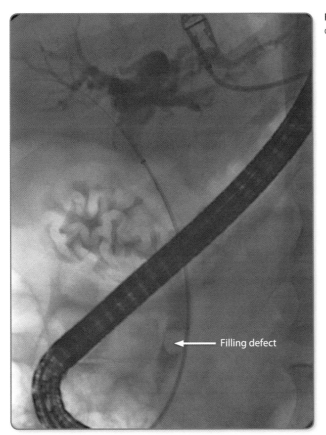

Figure 1.14 ERCP demonstrating ductal stones.

← Filling defect

paper or in the pan after defaecation. A sentinel pile (a skin tag distinct from a haemorrhoid) is a common marker of an anal fissure and also prognosticates that it may be difficult to manage conservatively.

82. C Fistula-in-ano

The discharge of fluid in this patient's case represents a fistula. Fistula-in-ano is a feature of the chronic stage of abscess formation and can occur due to simple cryptoglandular infection or trauma, Crohn's disease tuberculosis, cancer or radiation. The external opening can be used to locate the internal opening by following Goodsall's rule. Approximately 90% of fistulae with an external opening anterior to the midline will open into the anal canal anteriorly (in a radial fashion). Fistulous openings posterior to the midline will follow a horseshoe shape to open posteriorly in the midline (**Figure 1.15**).

83. J Teratoma

Testicular neoplasms commonly present following a minor scrotal injury. The patient who self-examines may feel a new lump which he attributes to the injury.

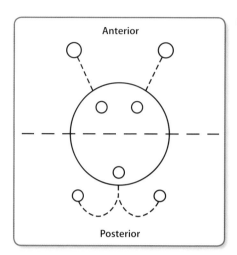

Figure 1.15 Goodsall's rule.

Commonly, the lesion is pre-existing and was previously too small or asymptomatic to be noticed in the absence of regular examination. A raised serum β-human chorionic gonadotropin (β-hCG) and α-fetoprotein is diagnostic of a testicular germ cell (non-seminomatous) tumour.

84. B Epididymal cyst

Epididymal cysts are benign, fluid-filled swellings in the head of the epididymis which do not usually require treatment. They are normally distinct from the testicle and transilluminate brightly.

85. F Idiopathic scrotal oedema

Acute idiopathic scrotal oedema is a relatively rare cause of an acute scrotum. It is characterised by a rapid onset of marked oedema (with or without erythema), without any tenderness. The child is normally apyrexial and all diagnostic tests are negative. The aetiology of this condition is unknown although helminth infection has been postulated as a cause.

86. D Excision of cyst

This patient is likely to have an epididymal cyst, although it may represent a more sinister lesion. Simple epididymal cysts are normally treated conservatively unless they change or the patient becomes symptomatic. In such cases surgery, in the form of excision, is recommended. Newer techniques to treat epididymal cysts have started to emerge including the use of sclerotherapy under ultrasound guidance.

87. F Immediate surgical exploration

This adolescent should be suspected to have a testicular torsion and merits immediate surgical exploration. The diagnosis is suspected on history and examination findings but should be confirmed by operation. If a viable testicle is found it should be untwisted and fixed in that position.

Classically a testicular torsion presents in infants and adolescents with sudden onset severe scrotal pain. The testicle may be tender and lying high in the scrotum. The chance of testicular salvage decreases as the duration of torsion increases. A torsion less than 6 hours is almost always viable whereas a torsion over 24 hours is never viable.

88. K Testicular vein embolisation

This patient has a varicocoele which is an abnormal dilation of the testicular vein due to defective valves, compression or obstruction. Approximately 98% develop on the left side because of the 90° angle of insertion of the testicular vein into the left renal vein. On the right the drainage is directly into the inferior vena cava. Examination findings are likened to a 'bag of worms'. When patients are symptomatic and desire treatment the most common method is by radiological embolisation of the testicular vein.

89. G Mittelschmerz

Mittelschmerz is mid-cycle lower abdominal or pelvic pain which can occur suddenly and may be present for several days. Diagnosis is one of exclusion whereby ultrasound scan normally reveals no abnormal findings or a trace of pelvic fluid.

90. F Mesenteric adenitis

The family history of inflammatory bowel disease is a distractor here as there are no gastrointestinal symptoms. This boy is likely to have mesenteric adenitis secondary to his recent upper respiratory viral illness. Mesenteric adenitis commonly mimics appendicitis but as this patient is hungry and thirsty, it can be reasonably safe to exclude appendicitis as a potential cause.

91. L Terminal ileal Crohn's disease

Crohn's disease can affect any part of the gastrointestinal tract from the mouth to the anus. The main symptoms of terminal ileal Crohn's disease are diarrhoea, abdominal pain and weight loss. The inflammation can lead to the development of a mass and malaise, lethargy, anorexia, nausea and vomiting may also feature.

92. D Decompression of tension pneumothorax

In this patient, the hyper-resonance and tracheal deviation is diagnostic of a tension pneumothorax. This occurs when the air leak into the pleural space increases to the point, where it pushes the mediastinum (including trachea) to the opposite hemithorax. There can be pressure on the cava with a massive decrease in cardiac output. The treatment here is emergency needle thoracostomy to decompress the thorax prior to insertion of a formal intercostal chest drain.

93. K Thoracotomy

In a trauma situation a positive pericardiocentesis is an indication for an emergency thoracotomy. Although a pericardiocentesis may have some benefit, it is essentially a diagnostic and temporizing procedure. The cause of the bleeding in the pericardial space needs to be addressed and this requires a thoracotomy. In the above patient's case, the positive focused assessment with sonography for trauma (FAST) scan for pericardial blood should have been enough to have mandated a thoracotomy, although the pericardial decompression may have been a life - saving measure.

94. H Laparotomy

Patients with a penetrating injury who are haemodynamically unstable require immediate operation. This includes those patients who are 'non-responders' and those who only transiently respond to fluid bolus administration. There should not be a delay for unnecessary investigations or interventions.

In junctional injuries (such as chest/abdomen) a decision must be made on which cavity to expose first. If at laparotomy there is no identified source of bleeding a thoracotomy should be performed (and vice versa). In the above patient's case, with exposed omentum the peritoneum has clearly been breached and the first course of action is to perform a laparotomy.

95. F 6

The Child–Pugh classification uses five variables (albumin, bilirubin, international normalised ratio, severity of ascites and encephalopathy), and each is scored between 1 (most normal) and 3 (most abnormal). The sum of the five scores generates the Child–Pugh score ranging from 5–15 (**Table 1.9**). The score corresponds to a Child–Pugh grade of A, B or C which can be used to classify the prognosis for the patient.

The patient in this question will score 1 for all of the above fields except for bilirubin (2). This gives a total score of 6 which is equivalent to Child–Pugh class A (**Table 1.10**).

Table 1.9 Child–Pugh score			
Measure	**1**	**2**	**3**
Albumin (g/L)	> 35	28–35	< 28
Ascites	None	Mild	Moderate/severe
Bilirubin (µmol/L)	< 34	34–50	> 50
Encephalopathy	None	Grade I–II	Grade III–IV
International normalised ratio (INR)	< 1.7	1.71–2.3	> 2.3

Table 1.10 Child–Pugh classification			
Points	**Class**	**1-year survival (%)**	**2-year survival (%)**
5–6	A	100	85
7–9	B	81	57
10–15	C	45	35

96. B 2

The patient has a modified Glasgow acute pancreatitis score of 1. This score is composed of eight criteria. It is used to predict severity, with a score >3 in the first 48 hours being predictive of severe pancreatitis.

The acronym **PANCREAS** can be used to remember the criteria:

Partial oxygen pressure <7.9 kPa

Age >55 years

Neutrophilia: WCC >15 x 10^9/L

Calcium <2.0 mmol/L

Renal: urea >16 mmol/L

Enzymes: lactate dehydrogenase >600 U/L

Albumin <32 g/L

Sugar: glucose >10 mmol/L

97. E 5

The Rockall scoring system (**Table 1.11**) uses the above criteria to identify patients at risk of adverse outcome following an upper gastrointestinal bleed. The clinical features (age, shock and comorbidity) and endoscopic findings (active bleeding and pathological cause) generates a score between 0 and 11.

Table 1.11 The Rockall scoring system				
Variable	**0**	**1**	**2**	**3**
Age	<60 years	60–79 years	>80 years	
Shock	None	SBP > 100 mmHg	SBP < 100 mmHg	
Comorbidity	None		Congestive heart failure Ischaemic heart disease Major morbidity	Renal/liver failure Metastatic cancer
Diagnosis	Mallory–Weiss	Others	Gastrointestinal malignancy	
Bleeding	None		Bleeding	

The Rockall score has been shown to be predictive of the risk of rebleeding and death. Those patients who score <3 have a good prognosis, whereas those with a score >8 have a higher risk of mortality.

98. C Calciphylaxis

Patients with end stage renal failure may develop calciphylaxis which is deposits of calcium in the small and medium sized vessels. These can present as painful plaques with surrounding purpura which can progress to ischaemic skin lesions with areas of necrotic skin. Necrotic components are typically dark bluish purple or completely black and leathery.

99. A Acanthosis nigricans

Acanthosis nigricans is a dermatological condition which presents with hyperpigmented, thickened skin, which is most marked over body flexures. It is associated with malignancy and in a study of 277 cases (Rigel et al. 1980) 56% had gastric carcinomas in 55.5%, 18% had another form of intra-abdominal malignancy and 27% had various other malignancies.

100. G Lentigo maligna

Lentigo maligna is a melanoma in situ which is normally found as a slow growing pigmented lesion on sun exposed areas. It is considered a precancerous lesion which grows slowly over many years. The lifetime risk of malignant transformation ranges from 2.2–4.7%.

101. C Amiloride

Amiloride (like spironolactone) is a potassium sparing diuretic which blocks the sodium channels in the distal convoluted tubules and collecting ducts, thereby inhibiting sodium reabsorption. Salt and water are lost in the urine, whereas potassium is retained and this may result in hyperkalaemia.

102. M Simvastatin

Statins are absolutely contraindicated in pregnancy because of the suspected risk to the fetus. As statins inhibit cholesterol production (which is required for fetal development) there is a risk of teratogenesis and the development of the vertebral defects, anal atresia, cardiac defects, tracheo-eosophageal fistula, renal anomalies and limb abnormalities (VACTERL) syndrome. However, other groups have suggested, there is no evidence that exposure to simvastatin increase the rate of congenital abnormalities in pregnant women.

103. L Noradrenaline

The main categories of adrenergic receptors relevant to vasopressor activity are the α_1-, β_1-, and β_2-adrenergic receptors and the dopamine (δ) receptors. Dopamine has varying effects on receptors depending upon the dose used (**Table 1.12**).

- α_1-adrenergic agonism leads to peripheral arteriolar vasoconstriction.
- β_1-adrenergic agonism leads to increased heart rate and force of contractility.
- β_2-adrenergic agonism leads to bronchial smooth muscle and skeletal muscle relaxation.
- (δ) dopaminergic agonism leads to increased renal blood flow at low doses. At higher doses there are also cardiac and vasoconstrictive effects.

Table 1.12 Inotropes and vasopressors				
	α_1	β_1	β_2	δ
Adrenaline	++	++	+	−
Noradrenaline	+++	+	−	−
Dopamine	++ (high dose)	++ (intermediate dose)	+	+ (low dose)
Dobutamine	+	+++	++	−

104. B α-Fetoprotein

Serum α-fetoprotein (AFP) can be used to diagnose, and guide the treatment of hepatocellular carcinoma (HCC). Normal serum values are <10 ng/mL, but they can be elevated in hepatitis to values as high as 100 ng/mL. In previously well individuals, a serum AFP > 400 ng/mL is diagnostic of HCC. However, in those with ongoing liver disorders (e.g. hepatitis) a value of > 4000 ng/mL is required to diagnose HCC.

AFP is useful in assessing the response to treatment for HCC. Following complete tumour removal, the AFP level should normalise. If it subsequently elevates, it suggests a tumour recurrence.

105. E Cancer antigen (CA) 19-9

This assay was originally developed to diagnose colorectal cancer, but in current practice it is more commonly used for patients with pancreatic cancer. The upper limit of normal for the CA19-9 assay is 37 U/mL and in the early stages of pancreatic cancer the blood levels are often normal, so it is not a useful screening test. The overall sensitivity of this assay is approximately 80% with a specificity of approximately 90%. When tumours generate blood levels of CA19-9 >1000 U/mL it is often an indication that the tumour is unfortunately unresectable.

106. M Human chorionic gonadotrophin

Three tumour markers are used in men with testicular germ cell tumours; the β subunit of human chorionic gonadotropin (β-hCG), α-fetoprotein (AFP) and lactate dehydrogenase (LDH). The most commonly used markers are AFP and β-hCG. AFP is never elevated in pure seminomas and β-hCG is only elevated in approximately a quarter of cases. AFP and β-hCG are both elevated in about 80% of non-seminomatous germ cell tumours (NSGCTs). LDH is not used as a diagnostic test but high levels are predictive of decreased survival.

107. A Duodenal atresia

Duodenal atresia is a failure of embryological development which results in the closure, or absence, of part of the duodenum. It occurs in 1 in 2500 live births and infants normally present with early onset of (commonly bilious) vomiting. The diagnosis of duodenal atresia can be confirmed by plain abdominal radiography or ultrasound which demonstrates the classical 'double bubble sign'. There is a significant association with Down's syndrome, given that approximately 20–40% of all infants with duodenal atresia have Down's syndrome and approximately 8% all infants with Down's syndrome have duodenal atresia. Correctional surgery is always necessary.

108. I Meconium ileus

Cystic fibrosis (CF) is an autosomal recessive disorder which presents with meconium ileus in 10–20% of patients. The highly viscous meconium can lead to intestinal obstruction which is suggestive of the diagnosis of CF. The majority of infants (90%) presenting with meconium ileus are subsequently diagnosed with CF.

109. E Hirschsprung's disease

Hirschsprung's disease is congenital aganglionosis of the distal colon as a consequence of abnormal fetal development and neural crest migration. The myenteric (Auerbach) plexus and the submucosal (Meissner) plexus are both affected which leads to decreased peristalsis in the affected segment. The anus is always involved and aganglionosis normally extends proximally for a short distance.

Hirschsprung's disease should be considered in a newborn with delayed passage of meconium, or a child with constipation since birth. Other symptoms include abdominal distension and vomiting. Most infants pass meconium by 24 hours and if there is none by 48 hours, a rectal examination should be performed. There may be explosive stools after an examining finger is gently placed in the rectum. Definitive diagnosis is normally made by performing a rectal suction biopsy.

110. C Forest plot

A Forest plot is a visual method used in meta-analysis to display the relative strength of treatment effects in multiple studies examining the same specific question. It normally has a left hand column containing the names of the studies (in chronological order) and a right hand column which displays the treatment effect as an odds ratio. A square with horizontal lines is used to represent the odds ratio and the confidence interval (this is numerically represented adjacent to the diagram). The size of each square represents its weight in the overall analysis (**Figure 1.16**).

A vertical line representing no effect (at odds ratio = 1) is plotted. A cumulative meta-analysis line is also plotted (below as a dotted line). The meta-analysed measure of effect is plotted as a diamond where the points represent the confidence intervals.

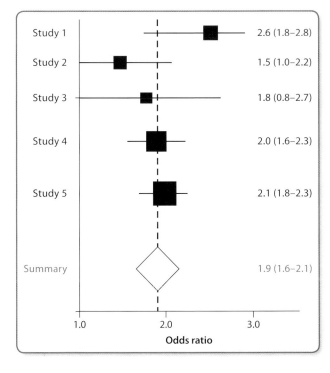

Figure 1.16 Forest plot.

111. H *p*-value

A type I error is a false positive. In statistical terms this means the test identifies a difference or a finding, when none actually exists. The rate of this error is noted as 'α', and is equivalent to the statistical significance.

In studies a *p*-value is quoted as the significance level, or the chance of a type I error. In layman's terms when interpreting a *p*-value it is best to think of it as the odds that the test would have produced the same result through chance alone.

112. F Likelihood ratio

A likelihood ratio (LR) is a measure of diagnostic accuracy and normally refers to a test or an investigation. When considering a clinical finding, the LR is the probability of that finding in patients with disease, divided by the probability of the same finding in patients without disease:

$$LR = \frac{\text{Probability of finding in patients with disease}}{\text{Probability of finding in patients without disease}}$$

For example, in patients with suspected diverticulitis, if the physical sign of 'left iliac fossa (LIF) tenderness' is present in 90% of patients with confirmed diverticulitis, and 30% without diverticulitis (i.e. because of urinary sepsis, pelvic inflammatory disease, etc.), then the LR for 'LIF tenderness' in detecting diverticulitis is 3.0 (90% divided by 30%).

A LR > 1 suggests strongly for the diagnosis of interest and the greater the number, the more convincingly the finding suggests that disease. LR < 1 argues against the diagnosis of interest and the closer to 0, the less likely the disease.

113. A Case–control study

There is a population of patients with an adverse outcome, and knowledge of the hypothesised risk factor. Although a longitudinal series would provide firm evidence of causal relationship, it would be possible to test his hypothesis by case-matching patients with, and without incisional hernias at 1 year postoperative, and constructing odds ratios relative to body mass index data in 2 x 2 tables.

114. F Meta-analysis

This describes an opportunity to perform a meta-analysis of available accrued trial data, with the cumulative numerical output being standard approach for meta-analysis.

115. E Longitudinal cohort series

This scenario describes an opportunity to demonstrate the value of rigorous, longitundinal data in adding to the evidence base. Often, data pertaining to 'real life' practice, and effectiveness, rather than overall efficacy data generated from randomised controlled trials, are highly useful and applicable to daily practice, and should not be overlooked in generating levels of evidence in guidelines and recommendations (**Table 1.13**).

Table 1.13 Examples of an evidence grading system and levels of recommendation, for use in developing clinical guidelines*

(a) Evidence grading: studies required for each level of evidence

Level	*Either* meta-analyses	*Or* systematic reviews	*Or* randomised controlled trials (RCTs)	*Or* Other
1++	√ (high quality)	√ (of RCTs only)	√ (if very low risk of bias)	–
1+	√ (well conducted)	√	√ (if low risk of bias)	–
1–	√	√	√ (if high risk of bias)	–
2++	–	√ (of case–control or cohort studies)	–	Case–control or cohort, if high quality, very low risk of confounding/bias, with high probability for causal relationship
2+	–	–	–	Case–control or cohort, if well conducted, low risk of confounding/bias, moderate probability for causal relationship
2–	–	–	–	Case–control or cohort, if high risk of confounding/ bias, high probability of no causal relationship
3	–	–	–	Case reports, case series
4	–	–	–	Expert opinion

(b) Levels of recommendation

Level	Studies required for each level of recommendation**
A	≥ 1 study at evidence level 1++ or Body of reports mainly at level 1+, with consistent results overall
B	Body of reports including evidence level 2++, with consistent results overall or Evidence extrapolated from reports at evidence level 1+/1++
C	Body of reports including evidence level 2+, with consistent results overall or Evidence extrapolated from reports at evidence level 2++
D	Reports at evidence level 3/ 4 or Evidence extrapolated from reports at evidence level 2+

*Based on the levels used by the Scottish Intercollegiate Guidelines Network (SIGN. Guideline 50: a guideline developer's handbook, revised edition. Edinburgh: SIGN, 2011. http://sign.ac.uk/pdf/sign50.pdf (last accessed October 2012)

** For recommendation levels A– C, studies must be directly applicable to the target population.

116. A χ^2 test

This scenario is going to compare two categorical groups (men, women) by a specific categorical outcome (readmission: yes/no). This requires a comparison of proportions in a 2 x 2 table. If numbers were very small, the Fisher's exact test should be used instead. Standard statistical programmes usually compute both test statistics in the appropriate setting, and the output advises which one should be applied based on variance.

117. E Mann–Whitney U test

In this scenario two categories of patients, laparoscopic and open surgery, are to be compared by a continuous outcome (which is unlikely to have a normal or parametric distribution). A non-parametric test comparing location of central tendency (median and interquartile range); the Mann-Whitney U test should be used. This is the non-parametric equivalent of the t-test. If data had been paired (i.e. patients matched by sex, tumour stage, and only varying by operative approach), then the Wilcoxon sign rank test would need to be used instead.

118. C Kruskal–Wallis test

This third scenario compares a continuous variable between four categories of patients. The continuous variable outcome is likely to exhibit highly skewed distribution. It is safest to assume the data is not normally distributed and use non-parametric testing. The Kruskal–Wallis test should be used unless the pain data are normally distributed. In such an unlikely situation, the ANOVA test should be used. The Kruskal–Wallis test may be thought of as the Mann–Whitney U test for more than three groups.

119. B Basal skull fracture

This man may have sustained significant trauma, possibly cumulatively, from head injuries some of which will have gone untreated/assessed. Trauma is the second most common cause of facial nerve palsy after Bell's palsy. Delayed paralyses can occur in the context of expanding haematomas and need not directly follow injury. The facial nerve is prone to injury at many sites along its course (**Figure 1.17**). Bhatoe (2007) provides a full review of trauma and cranial nerve injuries.

120. H Ramsay Hunt syndrome

Ramsay Hunt syndrome is essentially 'shingles' of the facial nerve, specifically the geniculate ganglion causing herpes zoster oticus. In this patient's case predisposing factors include immunocompromise (as a result of chemotherapy for malignant disease). It is often preceded by a painful rash around the external auditory meatus and is managed with steroids and antiviral medications.

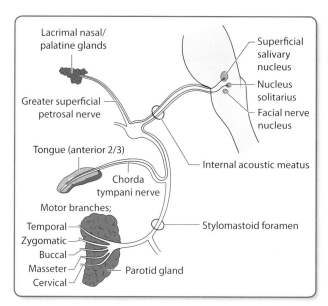

Figure 1.17 Course of the facial nerve, demonstrating the vulnerability of the nerve at many points.

121. I Squamous cell carcinoma

This scenario describes a typical patient predisposed to squamous cell carcinoma and (having had one already diagnosed and treated) this predisposes to another, particularly if the risk factors remain unmodified. It is an extremely rare tumour, when the primary site is the temporal canal, however, in this case, it may equally be secondary foci of the original tumour. Equally, it may arise as a clinically similar entity, through extension of a simple squamous carcinoma of the skin. It may also occur as a sequelae of chronic otitis media. Irrespectively, it is the most likely diagnosis in this man's case.

122. B Dermatofibroma

The differential diagnosis of this relatively common skin lesion is a malignant melanoma with excisional biopsy necessary for certainty. They are most common on the lower limbs in young–middle aged women, and tend to be small, brown or dark pink, pigmented hemispheric nodules, with a firm woody feel, mobile over the deep tissues. Some aetiological theories associate them with minor traumas such as insect bites. However, the more likely factor is sun exposure in this particular scenario. Other theories suggest they are the result of an immunoreactive process, with normal dermal dendritic cells being the initiators.

123. C Dermoid cyst

Dermoid cysts are smooth, spherical swellings which are soft, fluctuant and non-tender. They may be congenital or acquired. They are deep to the skin, differing from lipomas (in that they are not within the fat layers), and from sebaceous cysts (in that they are not attached to the skin). Acquired dermoid cysts usually follow trauma with implantation of skin into subcutaneous tissues (e.g. seen on fingers). Congenital lesions are due to developmental inclusion of epidermis along lines of fusion of skin dermatomes, and are therefore most commonly found at the corners of the brows, the midline of the nose, and the midline of the neck and trunk. Full excision, with extent established on imaging, is the only treatment (but is only necessary if the patient so wishes).

124. D Keratoacanthoma

Keratoacanthomas are found on sun-exposed skin, and tend to be more common in men. They are dome-shaped, with a keratin-containing central crater which is the only pigmented part. This aids the main differentiation from a rapidly growing melanoma. They may be further confused for a squamous cell carcinoma, with similar distributions, but the pit is characteristic. In the elderly, where there is a higher index of suspicion of the squamous cell differential, excision is generally advised. However, keratoacanthomas may regress as rapidly as they have grown.

125. I Warthin's tumour

There is a wide differential of tumours arising in the parotid gland. The lack of facial nerve involvement in this patient's case points to a benign process. Facial nerve involvement is suggestive of malignancy, but it can also occur in inflammatory processes (such as parotitis, **Figure 1.18**). By the man's age, and with smoking as a risk factor, a Warthin's tumour is the most likely diagnosis. This is the second most common of all tumour types. 80% of salivary tumours arise in the parotid gland, and of these, 80% are benign, with 80% of these being benign pleomorphic adenomas. With only a superficial component involved, the surgery may be limited to superficial parotidectomy; if deeper, the facial nerve should be preserved between resection of both lobes.

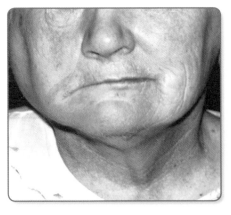

Figure 1.18 Right parotitis causing swelling and nerve palsy.

126. H Sjögren's syndrome

In this autoimmune syndrome (more common in women) swelling may be unilateral or bilateral, affecting any, or all salivary gland(s). The syndrome is diagnosed in the presence of at least two of a triad of (i) keratoconjunctivitis sicca, (ii) xerostomia and (iii) associated connective tissue disorders (such as rheumatoid arthritis, lupus, polymyositis, and scleroderma). Without the latter, it is known simply as Sjögren's disease. Patients with salivary calculi may also be reluctant to eat, because of painful secretory functions. In Sjögren's, patients are at a significantly increased risk of secondary lymphoma. The disease process is mediated through B-cell hyper-reactivity. Steroids are routinely used as systemic treatment.

127. B Frey's syndrome

Frey's syndrome is a complication of parotidectomy. This patient may have had only a superficial parotidectomy, with recurrent disease, however, he has developed Frey's syndrome postoperatively. Here increased sweating occurs on the facial skin when eating, because of reinnervation of divided sympathetic nerves to the facial skin by fibres of the secretomotor branch of the auriculotemporal nerve. It can affect up to 100% of patients postoperatively, but only 40% patients comment if questioned, and only 10% offer a spontaneous complaint, according to De Bree et al. (2007).

128. E Incarcerated inguinal hernia

This patient probably has an incarcerated inguinal hernia. Although femoral hernias are more common in women than in men (4:1 ratio), inguinal hernias remain more common among women than femoral hernias.

Full assessment should follow, and if the hernia remains irreducible with tight incarceration, it may be impossible to differentiate (between femoral and inguinal) prior to surgery. In such instances an inguinal approach would allow primary repair of either type of hernia.

129. D Hydrocele

This child probably has a hydrocele, made obvious by an increase in intra-abdominal fluid from his recent viral illness. The diagnosis implies the presence of an unobliterated/patent processus vaginalis, so, allowing fluid to track down. In infants, hydroceles are considered normal until such time that the processus has obliterated. Up to 90% show spontaneous resolution; however, they often remain asymptomatic, and can occur for a first time later in childhood, usually precipitated by such an event. These patients will require an operation for the processus to be ligated and the distal sac emptied.

130. G Inguinal lymphadenopathy

This man probably has inguinal lymphadenopathy – possibly resultant from insect bites on his distal limb, or another tropical illness. The history is inconsistent with a hernia or hydrocele, being tender, non-reducible, but appearing to have an upper margin and no cough impulse. Clinical lymphadenopathy requires full assessment, with a wide range of differential diagnoses – not infrequently excisional biopsy will be required to make a definitive diagnosis.

131. D Crohn's disease

The differential here is between an infective colitis, a distal colitis, and Crohn's disease. Given the mass, Crohn's disease is the most likely. Crohn's disease presents initially with bleeding in around 30% of cases, although it is relatively uncommon in purely terminal ileal disease. In patients with colonic Crohn's disease, bleeding is present in around 50%, and the other features of this patient's presentation suggest a colitic element. The palpable mass is typically caused by matted, thickened loops of small bowel. Typical radiological appearances can be seen in **Figure 1.19**. In the first instance, this patient should have endoscopic examination to allow histological diagnosis and systemic treatment with intravenous steroids. In more subtle presentations than this one, at colonoscopy, multiple biopsies should be taken anyway, as microscopic disease may be present, whereas appearing macroscopically normal. Surgical treatment would be considered in cases refractory to medical treatment with or without element of obstruction.

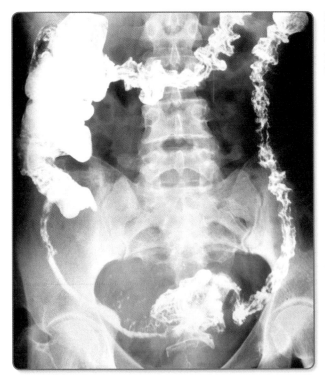

Figure 1.19 Crohn's disease on imaging. Typical stricturing with 'string sign' in a patient who presented clinically with a mass, from matted, inflamed bowel.

132. F Gastric carcinoma

The differential diagnosis here is between ischaemic colitis (smoking, non-tender abdomen) and gastric carcinoma. Given the background of weight loss, and melaena, gastric cancer is more likely. A further clue is provided by the possible evolving gastric outlet obstruction. Malignancy accounts for only 4% upper gastrointestinal (GI) bleeding, with peptic ulceration (any site, stomach or duodenum) collectively responsible for 35%.

In this case, it is the general malaise and weight loss that gives the clue to malignancy, although even an advanced, benign ulcer can lead to a degree of outlet obstruction. If the patient is haemodynamically stable, upper GI endoscopy should be carried out within the first 24 hours of admission. This will likely provide the diagnosis (visually and through biopsy of tissue) and will aid risk stratification for further/ongoing bleeding (depending on the nature of the lesion found). Malignant bleeding can be significant, and endoscopically difficult to control. Techniques such as argon coagulation, radiological embolisation or surgical intervention should be considered in relation to the patient's clinical condition and staging.

133. J Oesophagitis

This is straightforward oesophagitis in a young patient. He is not systemically unwell (as a patient with Boerhaave's syndrome would now have become) and the presentation is not acute enough for a Mallory–Weiss tear. The bleeding in this case is likely to be trivial, but treatment with proton pump inhibitor is warranted and endoscopic examination is required. In a patient who presents with systemic compromise, or symptoms of mediastinitis, a water soluble contrast swallow/CT should be arranged to define a Boerhaave's syndrome. This diagnosis can be difficult to make and requires a high index of suspicion. Pain can occur anywhere from neck to abdomen, and surgical emphysema may be revealed on examination of the neck. Hydrothorax, pneumothorax, or pneumomediastinum may be seen on chest X-ray or CT (**Figure 1.20**). If investigations prove negative, but the index of suspicion is still high, a careful flexible oesophagoscopy may be performed.

134. F Metronidazole

In this scenario, optimal cover for both gram negatives and anaerobes is required, with a fairly aggressive regimen appropriate to the aim of conservative management. Metronidazole is an essential component of therapy, whether a cephalosporin, or gentamicin with or without amoxycillin, is chosen in addition. Although antibiotics are clearly crucial in a conservative treatment plan, they must also be instituted prior to any operation, with a well-documented impact on reducing viable bacterial populations in peritonitis. In any such scenario, an active plan for repeated assessment is essential, with operative intervention if an inadequate improvement is seen.

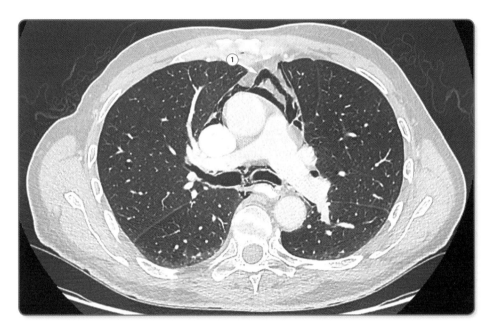

Figure 1.20 CT evidence of pneumomediastinum ⓵. This patient sustained an endoscopic perforation – and subsequent scan shows extensive mediastinal air early in the clinical course: this was not apparent on chest X-ray.

135. A Benzylpenicillin

This clinical scenario is representative of necrotising fasciitis and requires appropriately aggressive management, as soon as a clinical diagnosis is made. Benzylpenicillin is essential in any mixed pathogen aggressive soft tissue infection as it provides baseline streptococcal cover. Clindamycin may be added, or used in true cases of penicillin allergy. However, the nature of such mixed organism soft tissue infection (predisposed to among intravenous drug abusers, people with diabetes and other patients with immunocompromise) requires early surgical assessment and debridement, clearing any non-viable tissue in the field. A best practice guide is summarised in Hasham et al. (2005).

136. G None

No prophylaxis is necessary according to NICE guideline CG64 (NICE; 2008). The question here is regarding the necessary steps towards the prevention of bacterial endocarditis. Although both acquired valvular heart disease, and prosthetic replacements both predispose to risk of endocarditis, current recommendations from NICE state that prophylaxis should not be given routinely to at risk groups. Rather, it should only be given if the operative site is considered to be infected.

137. I RTS

The RTS (revised trauma score) is a tool with high interuser reliability, and is used to assess rapidly the risk of fatality in a trauma setting. It is simple to use and based only on Glasgow Coma Scale, systolic blood pressure and respiratory rate. A threshold of RTS < 4 is used to differentiate those patients requiring higher levels of care (**Table 1.14**).

Any one low-score parameter is enough to warn of a potentially adverse outcome.

The injury severity score (ISS), is a much more complex tool, whereby six body areas are assessed in full (requiring clinical assessment/radiology) and a score applied to predict outcome. It is an older instrument, originally described by Baker et al. (1974), with recent modifications. A useful summary of all trauma scores is also presented in Baker et al. (1974).

Table 1.14 Revised trauma score			
Glasgow Coma Scale	Systolic blood pressure (mmHg)	Respiratory rate (breaths per minute)	Coded value
13–15	> 89	10–29	4
9–12	76–89	> 29	3
6–8	50–75	6–9	2
4–5	1–49	1–5	1
3	0	0	0

138. E METS

This case would be ideal for functional assessment to quantify risk. The metabolic equivalent task score (METS) is a simple tool, devised to ascertain operative risk from activities of daily living which the patient routinely performs; the scores are set out in **Table 1.15**. If the patient is unable to achieve four METS, he may be considered high risk, in relation to the oxygen delivery capacity of his physiology. This assessment does depend on patient history, and anaesthetists often prefer simply observing a patient climb some flights of stairs. CPEX would be ideal for this patient,

Table 1.15 METs score	
METs score	Activity
1	Eat and dress, walk indoors around the house
2	Walk a block on the level, do light work around the house
4	Climb a flight of stairs/walk uphill, heavy domestic work, run short distance
6	Moderate recreational activities, e.g. dancing, golf
10	Strenuous sports, e.g. swimming

but his assessment will be limited by his comorbid arthritis, which would lead to underestimation of his physiological fitness. A helpful review of cardiopulmonary exercise testing is given in Hennis et al. (2011).

139. J SAPS II

Simplified acute physiology score II (SAPSII) is directly correlated to the risk of mortality in the intensive care patient, based on 14 biological and clinical parameters measured during the first 24 hours in intensive therapy unit (Le Gall et al. 1984). It was revised in 1993 based on a large multicentre study. It should be emphasised that these systems are only tools, and modifications to the 'results', require to be contextualised in patient populations. This particular tool is based on respiratory function, coagulation, liver function, blood pressure, Glasgow Coma Score, and renal function. The multiple organ dysfunction score (MODS) is less directly correlated with mortality risk, but various modifications of it exist so that this may be done.

140. A Elemental diet

An elemental diet is employed if there is limited digestive capacity (e.g. reduced gut area for absorption, or loss of enzymes). These diets contain nitrogen as oligopeptides which are more easily absorbed than free amino acids. It does induce a high osmotic load on the gut, and further 'dumping syndrome' type diarrhoea may evolve. However, this woman requires some form of supplementation, and without any obstruction or loss of gut function, there is no indication for feeding via a tube, or the parenteral route. A modular diet targets one particular group of nutrients which is missing from the diet.

141. I Total parenteral nutrition via Hickman/central line

This man essentially has intestinal failure, and the three essential elements of fistula management apply:

- Elimination of sepsis (drainage as required/antimicrobials)
- Gut rest
- Nutrition

With underlying Crohn's disease, it is unlikely that this lesion will heal spontaneously, particularly given the high output state. In order to approach surgery with the maximal chances of success, it is important to optimise his nutritional state. This may take a prolonged period of time. The gut is unsuitable for all the nutritional supplementation required because this will further drive the output. Therefore, parenteral nutrition should be instigated; as a long course is required, a tunnelled long line should be placed (to reduce the risk of peripheral line sepsis). This patient may be a candidate for home total parental nutrition until such time that definitive operative intervention is appropriate. There is evidence that supplemental enteral support is of additional benefit, with theoretical benefits because of effects on gut mucosa, but it cannot be relied upon in this case.

142. E Enteral feeding via surgically sited jejunostomy

The enteral route should be used for this patient's nutrition. Given the pylorus-preserving nature of his resection, some might be tempted to initiate early nasogastric feeding. However, this would mean feeding upstream from his pancreatic anastomosis, and distal enteric anastomoses; in order to optimise healing, feeding should take place downstream from the at-risk areas. Provocation of pancreatic enzymes can also thus be avoided. Further, delayed gastric emptying is recorded in a significant number of such procedures.

Chapter 2

Breast surgery

Questions: SBAs

For each question, select the single best answer from the five options listed.

1. A 25-year-old woman presents with a highly mobile, discrete lump in the outer aspect of her left breast.

   What is the most likely diagnosis?

   A   Breast carcinoma
   B   Ductal ectasia
   C   Duct papilloma
   D   Fibroadenoma
   E   Phyllodes tumour

2. A 28-year-old woman is diagnosed with a 4.5 cm fibroadenoma after attending the breast clinic.

   What is the most appropriate management?

   A   Mastectomy and axillary node sampling
   B   Neoadjuvant chemoradiotherapy
   C   Reassurance
   D   Simple excision
   E   Tamoxifen

3. A 46-year-old woman has a presumed fibroadenoma excised and the pathology report shows that the entire lesion consists of glands with very little intervening stroma.

   What is the most likely diagnosis?

   A   Breast cancer
   B   Hamartoma
   C   Lactating adenoma
   D   Phyllodes tumour
   E   Tubular adenoma

4. A 38-year-old woman undergoes a mammogram which is reported as showing a circumscribed area made up of soft and lipomatous tissue, surrounded by a thin radiolucent zone.

   What is the most likely diagnosis?

   A   Diabetic mastopathy
   B   Ductal papilloma
   C   Hamartoma
   D   Phyllodes tumour
   E   Pseudoangiomatous stromal hyperplasia of the breast

5. A 39-year-old woman presents to the breast outpatient clinic complaining of persistent nipple discharge. Examination reveals no mass lesion in either breast but bloodstained discharge from a single duct.

   What is the most appropriate initial investigation?

   A   CT of chest, abdomen and pelvis
   B   Ductography
   C   Mammogram
   D   Nothing else required
   E   Ultrasound of the breasts

6. A 38-year-old woman present with bloody nipple discharge. Examination reveals blood stained discharge from a single duct and but no other abnormality. Mammography is also reported as normal. The patient does not wish to have any further children.

   What is most appropriate management?

   A   Bilateral total duct excision
   B   Ductoscopy
   C   Mastectomy
   D   Reassurance only
   E   Total duct excision

7. A 67-year-old woman presents with a creamy discharge from her left nipple which has a slit-like appearance. There is no associated underlying mass.

   What is the most likely diagnosis?

   A   Duct ectasia
   B   Ductal papillomas
   C   Periductal mastitis
   D   Phyllodes tumour
   E   Physiological

8. A 45-year-old woman is involved in a road traffic accident but has no serious
    injuries, because she was wearing a seatbelt. She later notices a lump in her left
    breast with associated with skin retraction, ecchymosis and erythema. Results of the
    fine-needle aspiration show anuclear fat cells often surrounded by histiocytic giant
    cells and foamy phagocytic histiocytes.

    What is the most likely diagnosis?

    A   Breast cancer
    B   Duct ectasia
    C   Fat necrosis
    D   Fibrocystic disease
    E   Poland's syndrome

9. A 52-year-old woman has a 2 cm breast cyst aspirated and then 3 months later
    develops a swelling at the same site. Examination reveals a palpable, tender
    2 cm mass in the upper outer quadrant of the right breast. She undergoes a repeat
    ultrasound which shows a smooth outline and no internal echoes or posterior
    enhancement.

    What is the most appropriate management?

    A   Core biopsy
    B   Lumpectomy
    C   Mastectomy
    D   Needle aspiration
    E   Reassurance

10. A 37-year-old woman has been reviewed at a genetics clinic with a family history of
    breast cancer and has been found to carry a *BRCA1* gene mutation.

    What is the recommended surveillance that she should be offered?

    A   Alternative yearly MRI and mammography
    B   Annual clinical examination
    C   Annual mammography
    D   Annual MRI
    E   Two-yearly MRI

11. A family history of breast cancer increases the chances of developing the condition.

    Which statement defines an 8% risk of breast cancer in patients aged 30–39 years
    old?

    A   One close relative diagnosed with average age <30 years
    B   Two close relatives diagnosed with average age <25 years
    C   Two close relatives diagnosed with average age <30 years
    D   Two close relatives diagnosed with average age <40 years
    E   Three close relatives diagnosed with average age <40 years

12. A family history of breast cancer increases the chances of developing the condition.

Which statement defines a 12% risk of breast cancer in patients aged 40–49 years old?

A One close relative diagnosed with average age <25 years
B Two close relatives diagnosed with average age <45 years
C Three close relatives diagnosed with average age <50 years
D Three close relatives diagnosed with average age <55 years
E Four close relatives diagnosed with average age <50 years

13. A 54-year-old woman, who is asymptomatic, has diffuse microcalcification on screening mammography and undergoes stereotactic excision of a focal area of 1 cm ductal carcinoma in situ with macroscopically clear margins.

What is the most appropriate management?

A Axillary lymph node dissection
B Axillary clearance
C No specific axillary treatment
D Radiotherapy to the axilla
E Sentinel lymph node biopsy

14. A 65-year-old woman undergoes breast conserving surgery for an area of microcalcification. The pathology report describes a clear margin of <2 mm on the medial aspect of the wide local excision specimen, which contained ductal carcinoma in situ only and no invasive malignancy.

What is the most appropriate management?

A Axillary clearance
B Mastectomy
C Re-excision of the medial margin
D Re-excision of the lateral and medial margins
E Sentinel lymph node biopsy

15. A 49-year-old woman is postmenopausal and has undergone a wide local excision for a minute area of ductal carcinoma in situ, which has been completely excised.

What is the most appropriate management?

A Adjuvant chemotherapy
B Clinical follow-up only
C Tamoxifen
D Three years of letrozole treatment
E Trastuzumab

16. Which of the following statements describes sentinel lymph node biopsy?

    A   A biopsy-positive axilla is an absolute contraindication to sentinel lymph node
        biopsy
    B   A greater number of lymph nodes are harvested than compared with
        a sample
    C   It is associated with high morbidity
    D   It is mandatory in all patients with breast cancer
    E   The presence of isolated tumour cells is of great prognostic significance

17. A 49-year-old woman is diagnosed with Paget's disease of the nipple.

    What is the most appropriate treatment?

    A   Excision of nipple–areolar complex
    B   Nipple areolar conserving recentralisation surgery
    C   Radiotherapy alone
    D   Six-monthly mammography follow-up
    E   Total duct excision

18. Which of the following statements describes tamoxifen?

    A   It can be given to all patients with breast cancer
    B   It has no associated risk of uterine cancer
    C   It reduces recurrence and mortality if given for 5 years in oestrogen receptor
        (ER) positive cancer
    D   Tamoxifen has only a benefit in ER-negative breast cancers
    E   There is no increased risk of thromboembolism

19. Which of the following statements describes the use of anthracyclines in the
    adjuvant treatment of breast cancer?

    A   A dose of 50 g/m^2 of epirubicin has been shown to be optimal
    B   Congestive cardiac failure is a rare but serious side effect
    C   Herceptin is an anthracycline
    D   No significant side effects are associated with use
    E   There are no long-term consequences of taking anthracyclines

20. A 59-year-old woman has undergone a wide local excision for an early breast
    cancer but is found to have six positive lymph nodes.

    What is the most appropriate management?

    A   Internal mammary chain radiotherapy
    B   Clinic follow-up only in 3 months
    C   Mastectomy
    D   Supraclavicular fossa radiotherapy
    E   Tamoxifen only

21. A 45-year-old woman has been diagnosed and treated for an early breast cancer.

What is the most appropriate management?

A   Annual mammography
B   Biennial breast MRI
C   Ipsilateral soft tissue mammography after mastectomy
D   Six-monthly mammography
E   Three-yearly mammography

22. Which of the following statements describes advanced breast cancer?

A   External beam radiotherapy in a single fraction of 80 Gy can treat painful bone metastases
B   Positron emission tomography with CT (PET-CT) should be used routinely in advanced breast cancer
C   Women and men with invasive adenocarcinoma of clinical stages 1, 2 and 3 are included
D   Women and men with invasive adenocarcinoma of clinical stage 4 (known metastatic disease) are included
E   Women and men with metastases to the breast from other primary tumours are included

23. A 26-year-old woman, who underwent a breast augmentation 4 years ago presents to the breast clinic complaining of slight discomfort and hardness to the breast. Examination confirms that the breast is firm and there is an easily palpable capsule.

Which grade of capsular contraction is described?

A   Grade I capsular contraction
B   Grade II capsular contraction
C   Grade III capsular contraction
D   Grade IV capsular contraction
E   Grade V capsular contraction

24. Which of the following statements describes features of mastalgia?

A   Bromocriptine is widely used because of its low number of side effects
B   Reassurance can be the most effective treatment
C   Reducing fat intake has not been shown to have any benefit to symptoms
D   Tamoxifen is licensed as treatment for mastalgia
E   The use of a pain chart does not give objective evidence

25. A 46-year-old woman, who is premenopausal and has long-standing type 1 diabetes, presents with a large mass within the left breast. A fine-needle aspiration is reported as showing 'sclerosing lymphocytic lobulitis.'

What is the most likely diagnosis?

A   Breast cyst
B   Carcinoma
C   Diabetic mastopathy
D   Fibromatosis
E   Pseudoangiomatous stromal hyperplasia of the breast

26. Trastuzumab (Herceptin) is used in the treatment of HER2-positive breast cancer.

Which of the following statements is false?

A   Trastuzumab is a monoclonal antibody
B   A left ventricular ejection fraction (LVEF) of 75% or less is a contraindication to trastuzumab treatment
C   Trastuzumab can be used in the treatment of advanced HER2-positive gastric and gastro-oesophageal tumours
D   Patients on trastuzumab treatment require their cardiac function to be assessed 3 monthly
E   The duration of trastuzumab treatment is 1 year for HER2-positive early invasive breast cancer

27. Which of the following statements describes trastuzumab (Herceptin) treatment in breast cancer?

A   Cardiac function should be assessed at start of treatment and again if there are further concerns
B   It can be given if the patient has angina pectoris
C   It is contraindicated if the left ventricular ejection fraction (LVEF) is <60%
D   It is given at 3-weekly intervals over the course of 1 year
E   It should be stopped if there is a 5% drop in LVEF

28. Which of the following statements best describes docetaxel treatment in breast cancer?

A   It does not cause neutropenia
B   It is an anthracycline
C   It is not indicated for use in anthracycline-resistant breast cancers
D   Its side effects include oedema, arthralgia and myalgia
E   It should not be given in human epidermal growth factor receptor-2 overexpression breast cancers

29. Which investigation is indicated in patients with breast cancer?

   A   CT is the gold standard if breast density precludes accurate mammographic assessment

   B   Fine-needle aspiration with oestrogen receptor/progesterone receptor status is not required

   C   MRI is appropriate if there is discrepancy (between examination and imaging) regarding disease extent

   D   MRI should not assess tumour size in breast conserving surgery for invasive lobular cancer

   E   Pretreatment axillary ultrasound should only be performed in early invasive cancer with palpable nodes

30. A 47-year-old woman undergoes wide local excision and sentinel lymph node biopsy. Histopathology shows a 6-mm, grade 1, invasive ductal carcinoma. One out of three lymph nodes are positive for metastasis.

What is the Nottingham prognostic index for this patient?

   A   2.12

   B   3.12

   C   3.2

   D   4.2

   E   5.2

Questions: EMIs

Theme: Adjuvant treatments

A   Anastrozole
B   Corticosteroids
C   Cyclophosphamide
D   Epirubicin
F   Exemestane
G   Gemcitabine

H   Methotrexate
I   Megestrol acetate
J   Radiation menopause
K   Tamoxifen
L   Vinorelbine

Instructions: For each of the following descriptions, choose the single most appropriate treatment from the list above. Each option may be used once, more than once or not at all.

31. This has no role in postmenopausal patients.

32. The main side effects are significant weight gain and increased risk of thromboembolic disease.

33. This is used to perform ovarian ablation but can lead to gastrointestinal side effects.

Theme: Cytotoxic chemotherapy drugs

A   Anastrozole
B   Corticosteroids
C   Cyclophosphamide
D   Epirubicin
E   Erythromycin
F   Exemestane

G   Gemcitabine
H   Hydrocortisone
I   Megestrol acetate
J   Radiation menopause
K   Tamoxifen
L   Vinorelbine

Instructions: For each of the following descriptions, choose the single most appropriate treatment from the list above. Each option may be used once, more than once or not at all.

34. The main side effects of this agent are mouth ulcers and cardiomyopathy.

35. This is an antimetabolite which can cause coronary spasm and hand-foot syndrome.

36. This is a vinca alkaloid.

Theme: Male breast disease

A   Epidermal inclusion cyst
B   Glomus tumour
C   Lipoma
D   Haematoma
E   Fat necrosis
F   Gynaecomastia
G   Pseudoangiomatous stromal
     hyperplasia

H   Mastitis
I   Klinefelter's syndrome
J   Breast carcinoma
K   Lymphoma
L   Myofibroblastoma

Instructions: For each of the following scenarios choose the single most likely answer from the list above. Each option may be used once, more than once or not at all.

37. An 89-year-old man presents with a breast lump. He undergoes excisional biopsy. The pathology shows spindle cells and hyalinised collagen.

38. A 47-year-old man presents with a right breast lump. It is round circumscribed 2 cm lesion. On ultrasound, it is hypoechoic and the 'claw' sign is present.

39. A 75-year-old man presents with a painful left breast. On examination, the breast is swollen and erythematous. Mammograms reveal unilateral left sided breast enlargement with skin and trabecular thickening.

Theme: Nottingham prognostic index (NPI)

A   1.12
B   2.24
C   3.24
D   3.55
E   4.45
F   5.4

G   5.62
H   6.5
I   6.52
J   7.4
K   7.42
L   8.72

Instructions: For each of the following descriptions, choose the single most likely value from the list above. Each option may be used once, more than once or not at all.

40. A 55-year-old woman diagnosed with a 2 cm, grade 3 invasive ductal carcinoma with two lymph nodes positive for metastatic disease.

41. A 45-year-old woman diagnosed with a 2.5 cm, grade 3 invasive ductal carcinoma with five lymph nodes positive for metastatic disease.

42. A 76-year-old woman diagnosed with a 1.2 cm, grade 1 invasive ductal cancer with three lymph nodes positive for metastatic disease.

Theme: Nottingham prognostic index (NPI)

A	1.24	G	5.13
B	2.24	H	6.43
C	3.24	I	6.96
D	4.5	J	7.21
E	4.55	K	7.43
F	5.1	L	8.76

Instructions: For each of the following descriptions, choose the single most likely value from the list above. Each option may be used once, more than once or not at all.

43. A 35-year-old woman diagnosed with a 2.5 cm, grade 2 invasive ductal carcinoma with two out of five lymph nodes positive for metastatic disease.

44. A 27-year-old woman diagnosed with a 1.2 cm, grade 1 invasive ductal carcinoma with zero out of three lymph nodes positive for metastatic disease.

45. A 72-year-old woman diagnosed with a 4.8 cm, grade 3 invasive ductal carcinoma with seven lymph nodes positive for metastatic disease.

Theme: Genetics

A	*BRCA*	G	*CDH1*
B	*BRCA2*	H	*CHEK2*
C	*TP53*	I	*MRE11A*
D	*PTEN*	J	*NBN*
E	*ATM*	K	*PALB2*
F	*BRIP1*	L	*STK11*

Instructions: For each of the following scenarios, choose the single most likely genetic mutation from the list above. Each option may be used once, more than once or not at all.

46. A 58-year-old male presents with a lump 1-cm superior to the left nipple. He is diagnosed with breast cancer, and genetic testing is carried out. What is the most common type of genetic mutation in male breast cancer?

47. A 27-year-old woman with Peutz–Jeghers syndrome is diagnosed with breast cancer. Which genetic mutation is likely to be present?

48. A 45-year-old woman with a past history of soft tissue sarcoma aged 25 years is diagnosed with breast cancer. Which genetic mutation is likely to be present?

Theme: Breast pathology

A   Primary angiosarcoma of the breast
B   Ductal carcinoma in situ
C   Invasive ductal carcinoma
D   Invasive lobular carcinoma
E   Lymphoma of the breast
F   Male breast cancer
G   Melanoma of the breast

H   Metastases to the breast
I   Paget's disease
J   Pregnancy associated breast cancer
K   Pseudoangiomatous stromal
    hyperplasia
L   Secondary angiosarcoma of the breast

Instructions: For each of the following descriptions, choose the single most likely condition from the list above. Each option may be used once, more than once or not at all.

49. This commonly presents with multifocal pattern and painless skin nodules and is most commonly associated with radiation and long-standing lymphoedema.

50. The main treatment is chemotherapy based with surgery usually performed to obtain tissue diagnosis only.

51. A 37-year-old woman presents with excoriation of the nipple and surrounding skin and is advised that treatment of this disease should always include excision of the nipple-areolar complex.

Theme: Benign breast disease

A   Accessory breast tissue
B   Breast hypoplasia
C   Duct ectasia
D   Fibroadenoma
E   Juvenile hypertrophy
F   Macrocysts
G   Mastalgia

H   Mastopathy
I   Mondor's disease
J   Papilloma of duct
K   Pseudoangiomatous stromal
    hyperplasia of the breast
L   Sclerosis

Instructions: For each of the following scenarios, choose the single most likely diagnosis from the list above. Each option may be used once, more than once or not at all.

52. A 35-year-old woman presents to the outpatient clinic with unilateral breast discomfort and normal mammography and ultrasound.

53. A 24-year-woman presents to the outpatient clinic with a smooth, mobile lump in the outer aspect of her left breast.

54. A 65-year-old woman, who is a non-smoker, presents with a creamy discharge from her right nipple and a slit-like appearance to the nipple which is new.

Theme: Benign breast disease

A   Accessory breast tissue
B   Breast hypoplasia
C   Duct ectasia
D   Fibroadenoma
E   Juvenile hypertrophy
F   Macrocysts
G   Mastalgia
H   Mastopathy
I   Mondor's disease
J   Papilloma of duct
K   Pseudoangiomatous stromal
      hyperplasia of the breast
L   Sclerosis

Instructions: For each of the following descriptions, choose the single most likely condition from the list above. Each option may be used once, more than once or not at all.

55. Histology reveals sclerosis lymphocytic lobulitis.

56. A 45-year-old woman is found on clinical examination to have a thickened palpable cord-like structure with associated erythema in her right breast.

57. Immunohistochemistry vascular markers are required to avoid the differential diagnosis of mammary angiosarcoma.

Theme: Benign breast conditions

A   Accessory breast tissue
B   Breast hypoplasia
C   Cysts
D   Fat necrosis
E   Juvenile hypertrophy
F   Lipomatous disease
G   Mastalgia
H   Mastopathy
I   Montgomery's glands
J   Papilloma of duct
K   Pseudoangiomatous stromal
      hyperplasia of the breast
L   Sclerosis

Instructions: For each of the following descriptions, choose the single most likely condition from the list above. Each option may be used once, more than once or not at all.

58. Histology is characterised by anucleate fat cells surrounded by histiocytic giant cells.

59. These glands can block, cause hard nodules on the periphery of the areolar.

60. Imaging can reveal a radiolucent lobulated mass which commonly occurs in the sixth decade.

Answers: SBAs

1. D Fibroadenoma

This 25-year-old patient has a history and examination findings classical of a fibroadenoma, which are benign breast lumps that are common in women in their late teens or early twenties. They are mostly solitary findings but can be multiple. They are commonly called a 'breast mouse' because of the fact that they are highly mobile. In older women, differentiating a fibroadenoma from breast cancer is a necessity.

2. D Simple excision

As this 28-year-old woman has a 4.5 cm fibroadenoma, excision of the fibroadenoma is recommended. This is advised for any fibroadenoma when the size is >4 cm, there are concerns on histopathology, the patient wishes surgical excision, or where it is causing cosmetic changes to the appearance of the breast tissue.

3. E Tubular adenoma

This 46-year-old patient has a tubular adenoma. Tubular adenomas are diagnosed when the entire lesion consists of glands with very little intervening stroma. Lactating adenomas are very similar but occur in pregnant or lactating women, and clearly this is an important differentiating point to be elicited from the patient's history. Tubular adenomas are treated in the same manner as fibroadenomas, so excision is recommended only when they are of a large size, if there are any histological concerns, or if the patient has strong wishes for surgical excision.

4. C Hamartoma

This is the classical mammographic description of a hamartoma, with an encased area on a mammogram surrounded by a radiolucent rim.

5. C Mammogram

This patient is >35 years old and first line investigation should be referral for an urgent mammogram to rule out an underlying malignancy as a cause for her nipple discharge after an appropriate history and clinical examinations have been done. Ultrasound scan with or without biopsy can be carried out once the mammogram has been performed. Ductography is painful and is not normally carried out in the outpatient setting due to this, so if it was required, it should probably be undertaken during an anaesthetic to ensure that the procedure is comfortably tolerated.

6. E Total duct excision

This 38-year-old woman has had a normal mammogram and the next appropriate management would be to discuss total duct excision as a surgical option. It means that in excising all the ducts, all pathology is likely to be excised and a diagnosis achieved. An underlying malignancy is less likely to be missed compared with microdochectomy, whereby only a single duct is excised, but the latter may be the more appropriate form of surgery in women, who may still wish to breast feed in the future, i.e. in the younger childbearing population.

7. A Duct ectasia

This 67-year-old woman has a likely diagnosis of duct ectasia due to the creamy discharge. The incidence of duct ectasia increases with age and is usually an asymptomatic lesion which is detected mammographically because of microcalcifications. A mammogram is therefore essential as part of the assessment. Mammary duct ectasia should not be confused with periductal mastitis which is associated with younger women who smoke – an important issue to be asked in the history. Physiological discharge is usually from multiple ducts and is green in colour, so if discharge can be expressed from the nipple at clinic this can greatly aid diagnosis.

8. C Fat necrosis

The most likely underlying diagnosis in this 45-year-old woman is fat necrosis, which is a benign, inflammatory process of the breast. It can be caused by trauma such as in this case or is associated with an underlying malignancy. It is therefore imperative that a full triple assessment is performed to ensure that an underlying malignancy is not missed.

9. D Needle aspiration

This 52-year-old woman has a recurrent simple breast cyst which requires repeat aspiration and, as long as there is no residual lump after aspiration, the patient can be reassured and followed up routinely. However, if a lump remains after aspiration then further imaging and biopsy are required, including mammography and cytology on the residual lump. If this occurs, surgeons must be suspicious of an underlying malignancy and a core biopsy of the underlying lump will be appropriate.

10. D Annual MRI

The NICE guideline CG41 (NICE; 2006) on the family history of breast cancer recommends an annual MRI for this 37-year-old *BRCA1* carrier. When the patient is referred to the breast clinic, a family history should always be undertaken to allow stratification of risk and referral to a genetics team may be warranted.

11. C Two close relatives diagnosed with average age <30 years

An 8% risk of breast cancer in patients aged 30–39 years old is defined by the NICE guideline CG41 (NICE; 2006) as a patient having had two close relatives diagnosed with the disease, with their average ages less than 30 years old.

12. E Four close relatives diagnosed with average age <50 years

A 12% risk of breast cancer in patients aged 40–49 years old is defined by the NICE guideline CG41 (NICE; 2006) as a patient having had four close relatives diagnosed whose average ages are less than 50 years old.

13. C No specific axillary treatment

No further treatment is required in this patient, who has undergone excision of a focal area of ductal carcinoma in situ (DCIS) with clear margins. According to the NICE guideline CG80 (NICE; 2009) treatment would only be advised if the patient was deemed to be at high risk. Significant risk factors include those with a clinically detected lump or widespread microcalcifications.

14. C Re-excision of the medial margin

This 65-year-old woman should be offered re-excision of the medial margin as the clear margin is less than 2 mm. A minimum margin of 2 mm of excision is recommended with pathological examination and the NICE guideline CG80 (NICE; 2009) recommends that re-excision of the involved margin should be offered after a frank discussion with the patient. Clearly the patient has to be advised that there is no guarantee the re-excision margin will be clear and further surgery may be required.

15. B Clinical follow-up only

This 49-year-old has undergone breast conservation surgery for a minute area of ductal carcinoma in situ (DCIS), which has been completely excised. Therefore, the NICE guideline CG80 (NICE; 2009) for early and locally advanced breast cancer advises that this patient requires no further adjuvant treatment. She will be recommended to have clinical follow-up only.

16. A A biopsy positive axilla is an absolute contraindication to sentinel lymph node biopsy

If the patient is found to have a clinically or biopsy positive axilla, i.e. the presence of palpable lymph nodes or lymph nodes proven to be positive histologically, then sentinel lymph node biopsy is not recommended. Instead, patients should be offered the gold standard of treatment which is level II or III axillary lymph node dissection. The presence of isolated tumour cells is currently grouped with node-negative disease. However, some studies have shown that this may be an adverse prognostic factor.

17. A Excision of the nipple–areolar complex

Paget's disease of the breast commonly presents with skin changes to the nipple with evidence of excoriation. As it is an uncommon disease, surgeons need to have a high suspicion for it to be diagnosed and treated correctly. Treatment, as in the case of this 59-year-old woman, should always include excision of nipple-areola complex. Mastectomy has been advocated as the gold standard of treatment in the past, however, breast-conserving surgery with irradiation also shows low recurrence rates.

18. C It reduces recurrence and mortality if given for 5 years in oestrogen receptor (ER) positive cancer

The Early Breast Cancer Trialists Collaborative Group (2011) has shown that in oestrogen receptor (ER)-positive disease, a 5-year course of treatment with tamoxifen significantly decreased recurrence rates for the first decade, and therefore it should be advised in this patient group.

19. B Congestive cardiac failure is a rare but serious side effect

The French Adjuvant Study Group (2003) suggests that adjuvant treatment should involve the use of anthracyclines at a selected dose, and that epirubicin at 100 mg/m^2 may be the standard of treatment that is to be recommended. Further studies have shown that cardiotoxicity and acute myeloid leukaemia are complications that can result after treatment with such drugs.

20. D Supraclavicular fossa radiotherapy

The NICE guideline CG80 (NICE; 2009) recommends that this 59-year-old patient should undergo supraclavicular fossa radiotherapy as she has early breast cancer and has had more than four positive lymph nodes removed.

21. A Annual mammography

The NICE guideline CG80 (NICE; 2009) recommends that patients with early breast cancer should undergo follow-up, which includes an annual mammogram. This should happen until the patient is eligible to enter the national breast screening programme. If the patient has undergone a mastectomy as part of their treatment, mammograms of the remaining soft tissue of the side that was operated on are not required. NICE also states that MRI should not be offered as a standard follow-up for patients with an early breast cancer.

22. D Women and men with invasive adenocarcinoma of clinical stage 4 (known metastatic disease) are included

The NICE guideline CG81 (NICE; 2009) that for patients with advanced breast cancer (i.e. those with known metastatic disease and therefore clinical stage 4), position emission tomography with CT (PET-CT) can be used to aid clarification on metastases if there are areas of suspicion on the liver or other parts of the body; PET-CT should not be routinely used in all cases at present. For bony metastases, radiotherapy can be used in a palliative setting and the dose in this situation would be 8 Gy in a single fraction, not 80 Gy.

23. C Grade III capsular contraction

This is a Grade III capsular contraction if the Baker classification system is used. Grade III has been defined as a firm breast on clinical examination. Other grades of capsular contraction following implant insertion for breast augmentation have been described ranging from class 1 to class IV but surprisingly it is only the latter, i.e. grade IV, which is associated with an unacceptable clinical appearance.

24. B Reassurance can be the most effective treatment

Breast pain is a very common symptom that is seen at breast clinics. The use of a pain chart can provide objective evidence as to the debilitating effects of the pain on the patient's lifestyle. Reassurance is the mainstay of treatment provided an underlying cancer has been excluded. All patients >35 years old should have a mammogram performed to exclude this.

25. C Diabetic mastopathy

This is a rare condition mainly occurring in premenopausal women. As in this 46-year-old woman, diabetic mastopathy is linked to having type 1 diabetes and can present with a single or multiple lumps within the breast. As other sinister pathology must be excluded, fine-needle aspiration must be undertaken and if diabetic mastopathy is confirmed, the pathology will be revealed as showing sclerosing lymphocytic lobulitis.

26. B A left ventricular ejection fraction (LVEF) of 75% or less is a contraindication to trastuzumab treatment

Trastuzumab is a recombinant humanised monoclonal antibody, which is selective for the human epidermal growth factor receptor 2 (HER-2). It can be used in both early and advanced HER2-positive breast cancer. It is used for a year in the early stages, or until recurrence, and can be used as long as it is controlling the disease in advanced cases.

Side effects include allergic reactions, flu-like symptoms, headaches, nausea, anorexia, abdominal pain, diarrhoea/constipation, tiredness, joint pain, numbness in the hands and feet and neutropaenia. Cardiac complications, such as congestive cardiac failure and cardiomyopathy, may occur. Therefore prior to commencing treatment cardiac function should be assessed. A left ventricular ejection fraction (LVEF) of 55% or less is a contraindication to trastuzumab treatment, as is poorly controlled hypertension, congestive cardiac failure, uncontrolled arrhythmias, angina pectoris requiring medication, significant valvular cardiac disease and evidence of transmural infarction on ECG.

27. D It is given at 3-weekly intervals over the course of 1 year

The NICE guideline CG80 (NICE; 2009) recommends that trastuzumab (Herceptin) should be prescribed to HER2-postive women with a diagnosis of early invasive breast cancer. Because of trastuzumab's significant cardiac side effects, all patients should undergo full cardiac assessment including an echocardiogram pre- and during treatment with the drug. Treatment should be ceased if left ventricular ejection fraction reduces by 10% or falls below 50%. All women should be aware of and counselled for the cardiac side effects prior to commencement of treatment.

28. D Its side effects include oedema, arthralgia and myalgia

Docetaxel is a taxane which is used in the adjuvant treatment of breast cancer, especially in the metastatic setting of anthracycline resistant breast cancers. The UK Taxotere as Adjuvant Chemotherapy Trial (TACT) trial (Ellis et al., 2009) showed that in the taxane arm, there were increased side effects from neutropenia and lethargy and other studies have demonstrated oedema, arthralgia and myalgia are side effects of its use.

29. C MRI is appropriate if there is discrepancy (between examination and imaging) regarding disease extent

MRI can be successfully used to define the extent of lobular carcinoma and to evaluate the extent of an early invasive breast cancer, if there are concerning differences between clinical examination and other imaging modalities. The axilla should always be staged with ultrasound scan, even if no nodes are clinically palpable, to give a full and accurate preoperative staging.

30. B 3.12

The Nottingham prognostic index (NPI) is calculated using the formula:

$$NPI = [0.2 \times S] + N + G,$$

Where:

S = size of the index lesion in cm

N = node status: 0 nodes = 1, 1–4 nodes = 2, >4 nodes = 3

G = grade of tumour

In this patient, S = 0.6, N = 2 and G = 1, therefore NPI = [0.2 × 0.6] + 2 + 1 = **3.12**.

Answers: EMIs

31. J Radiation menopause

The aim of inducing a radiation menopause in breast cancer patients is to reduce the levels of the hormone oestrogen. This can be achieved by a process called ovarian ablation which is carried out either operatively (by laparoscopic or open oophorectomy) or through a short course of radiotherapy to the pelvis (to avoid gastrointestinal side effects) and is not indicated in postmenopausal patients. Hormonal therapy can also induce this.

32. I Megestrol acetate

Progesterones (e.g. megestrol acetate, medroxyprogesterone) have an anti-oestrogenic effect, but the complications associated with their use include significant weight gain and the increased risk of deep vein thrombosis or pulmonary emboli.

33. J Radiation menopause

Ovarian ablation can be achieved either operatively (by laparoscopic or open oophorectomy) or through a short course of radiotherapy to the pelvis (to avoid gastrointestinal side effects) and is not indicated in postmenopausal patients.

34. D Epirubicin

Epirubicin is an example of the group of drugs classed as anthracyclines, whose main side effects are mouth ulcers and cardiomyopathy.

35. G Gemcitabine

The antimetabolite class of drugs, e.g. methotrexate and gemcitabine, have the main side effects of coronary spasm and hand-foot syndrome.

36. L Vinorelbine

Vinorelbine belongs to the class of drugs called vinca alkaloids. Anastrozole and exemestane are both aromatase inhibitors and cyclophosphamide is classified as an alkylating agent. Epirubicin is an anthracycline.

37. L Myofibroblastoma

Myofibroblastoma is a rare benign stromal tumour generally found in elderly males. The pathogenesis is uncertain. Pathology shows spindle cells and hyalinised collagen. Excisional biopsy is adequate treatment and although these tumours may recur they rarely undergo malignant transformation.

38. A Epidermal inclusion cyst

Epidermal inclusion cyst is a dermal lesion. They are usually round, circumscribed, and typically range in size from 1–5 cm. The cysts contain laminated keratin with a wall of epidermis. On ultrasound, they are hypoechoic. The claw sign is a sonographic feature where the skin is compressed posteriorly and an echogenic curvilinear line from the skin is seen posteriorly along with posterior acoustic enhancement.

39. H Mastitis

Mastitis is an infection of the breast tissue. It is typically unilateral and may lead to abscess formation. On mammography skin and trabecular thickening is seen. With an abscess, an irregular mass +/– calcifications may be seen. It can be difficult to differentiate from malignancy. Treatment is with antibiotics +/– percutaneous drainage. In some cases, surgical excision of the abscess and involved duct may be required.

40. F 5.4

The Nottingham prognostic index (NPI) is calculated using the formula:

$$[0.2 \times S] + N + G$$

Where:

S is the size of the index lesion in centimetres

N is the number of lymph nodes involved: $0 = 1$, $1–3 = 2$, $>3 = 3$

G is the grade of tumour: Grade I $= 1$, Grade II $= 2$, Grade III $= 3$

In this patient $S = 2$, $N = 2$ and $G = 3$; therefore, the NPI is calculated as: $(0.2 \times 2) + 2 + 3 = 5.4$

41. H 6.5

The Nottingham prognostic index (NPI) is calculated using the formula:

$$[0.2 \times S] + N + G$$

Where:

S is the size of the index lesion in centimetres

N is the number of lymph nodes involved: $0 = 1$, $1–3 = 2$, $>3 = 3$

G is the grade of tumour: Grade I $= 1$, Grade II $= 2$, Grade III $= 3$

In this patient $S = 2.5$, $N = 3$ and $G = 3$; therefore, the NPI is calculated as: $(0.2 \times 2.5) + 3 + 3 = 6.5$

42. C 3.24

The Nottingham prognostic index is calculated using the formula:

$$[0.2 \times S] + N + G$$

Where:

S is the size of the index lesion in centimetres

N is the number of lymph nodes involved: 0 =1, 1–3 = 2, >3 = 3

G is the grade of tumour: Grade I = 1, Grade II = 2, Grade III = 3

In this patient S = 1.2, N = 2 and G = 1; therefore, the NPI is calculated as: (0.2 × 1.2) + 2 + 1 = **3.24**

43. D 4.5

The Nottingham prognostic index is calculated using the formula:

$$[0.2 \times S] + N + G$$

Where:

S is the size of the index lesion in centimetres

N is the number of lymph nodes involved: 0 = 1, 1–3 = 2, >3 = 3

G is the grade of tumour: Grade I = 1, Grade II = 2, Grade III = 3

In this patient S = 2.5, N = 2 and G = 2; therefore, the NPI is calculated as: (0.2 × 2.5) +2 + 2 = **4.5**

44. B 2.24

The Nottingham prognostic index is calculated using the formula:

$$[0.2 \times S] + N + G$$

Where:

S is the size of the index lesion in centimetres

N is the number of lymph nodes involved: 0 = 1, 1–3 = 2, >3 = 3

G is the grade of tumour: Grade I = 1, Grade II = 2, Grade III = 3

In this patient S = 1.2, N = 1 and G = 1; therefore, the NPI is calculated as: (0.2 × 1.2) + 1 + 1 = **2.24**

45. I 6.96

The Nottingham prognostic index is calculated using the formula:

$$[0.2 \times S] + N + G$$

Where:

S is the size of the index lesion in centimetres

N is the number of lymph nodes involved: 0 = 1, 1–3 = 2, >3 = 3

G is the grade of tumour: Grade I = 1, Grade II = 2, Grade III = 3

In this patient S = 4.8, N = 3 and G = 3; therefore, the NPI is calculated as: (0.2 × 4.8) + 3 + 3 = **6.96**

46. B *BRCA2*

10% of male breast cancer patients will carry the *BRCA2* gene.

47. L *STK11*

Peutz–Jeghers syndrome is an autosomal dominant condition. The carrier of the gene *STK11*, a tumour suppressor gene, develops hamartomatous polyps and mucocutaneous lesions. They are at higher risk not only of gastrointestinal tumours, but also breast, lung and ovarian tumours also.

48. C *TP53*

TP53 gene abnormalities cause Li-Fraumeni syndrome. Carriers develop sarcomas and cancers of the breast, brain and adrenal glands. Leukaemia, lymphoma and adrenocortical carcinoma are also seen in this syndrome.

49. L Secondary angiosarcoma of the breast

Angiosarcoma of the breast is rare. Secondary angiosarcomas usually present as pain-free skin lesions which are dark in colour. Malignant melanoma is a differential diagnosis which must be considered and excluded in such patients. Risk factors which may be linked with secondary angiosarcomas are radiation and chronic lymphoedema.

50. E Lymphoma of the breast

Primary breast lymphoma is a cause of 0.14% of all breast cancers and <2% of all non-Hodgkin's lymphomas. Patients usually present in their mid to late forties and surgery is really only used to provide adequate tissue to allow a diagnosis to be made and in turn to allow treatment to be commenced.

51. I Paget's disease

This 37-year-old woman has a diagnosis of Paget's disease where excision of the nipple areolar is the advised treatment option. There is still an ongoing debate surrounding the need for mastectomy, as breast-conserving surgery surgery combined with radiotherapy have been shown to have acceptable recurrence rates. Obviously both surgical options should be discussed with the patient. As in this scenario, Paget's can present with excoriation of the nipple causing an itching or burning irritation.

52. G Mastalgia

Breast pain is a common symptom that is referred to specialist breast clinics. Reassurance is the mainstay of treatment provided an underlying cancer has been excluded as in this patient, who has undergone a mammogram and ultrasound scan. All patients >35 years old should undergo a mammogram to exclude an underlying malignancy.

53. D Fibroadenoma

This 24-year-old woman has a likely fibroadenoma which has the colloquial name of a 'breast mouse' because of its increased mobility in the breast. These lumps are common in younger women and unless they are >4 cm, have underlying suspicious features or the patient wishes excision, can generally be left alone.

54. C Duct ectasia

This 65-year-old woman has duct ectasia with creamy discharge from a slit-like nipple. Duct ectasia is found with increasing incidence with age and is usually an asymptomatic lesion. It is detected mammographically because of microcalcifications. Mammary duct ectasia is commonly mistaken for periductal mastitis, but the important differentiating factor which should be elicited from the history is that periductal mastitis is associated with younger women who smoke.

55. H Mastopathy

This mainly occurs in premenopausal females and males with a chronic history of type 1 diabetes. It can present with one or multiple hard lumps within the breasts. Histology reveals sclerosing lymphocytic lobulitis.

56. I Mondor's disease

This is a classical description of Mondor's disease, which results from inflammation of a breast vein leading to erythema of the overlying skin and an underlying hard structure which is felt on examination and is in keeping with the vein being palpable. It can usually be treated conservatively with analgesics and anti-inflammatories and generally never affects the upper, inside aspect of the breast.

57. K Pseudoangiomatous stromal hyperplasia of the breast

Pseudoangiomatous stromal hyperplasia (PASH) of the breast is commonly found incidentally within breast biopsies which are being undertaken for the diagnosis of other conditions such as malignancy. The aetiology of PASH remains uncertain and immunohistochemical markers are required for diagnosis as other conditions can mimic it without full histological examination.

58. D Fat necrosis

The most likely underlying diagnosis in this 45-year-old women is fat necrosis. Fat necrosis of the breast is a benign, inflammatory condition. It can be caused by trauma, such as in this case, or associated with an underlying malignancy. It has a distinct pathological entity which makes diagnosing it clear.

59. I Montgomery's gland

This is a classical description of a prominent Montgomery's gland which produces fluid during breastfeeding to moisten the nipple. These glands can be susceptible to infection but, unless this is the case or they are symptomatic for other reasons, then most patients just require reassurance and an explanation for their presence.

60. F Lipomatous disease

This radiological description is of a lipoma which commonly present in women in their fifties and, as such, carcinoma must be excluded. Small carcinomas can masquerade as lipomas so triple assessment in the form of history and examination, radiological assessment and biopsy must be undertaken to ensure that an underlying cancer is not missed.

Chapter 3

Colorectal surgery

Questions: SBAs

For each question, select the single best answer from the five options listed.

1. A 75-year-old man, 2 years postradiation therapy for prostate cancer, presents to the outpatient clinic with anaemia and tenesmus. Flexible sigmoidoscopy reveals mucosal pallor and vascular telangiectasia.

   What is the most likely diagnosis?

   A   *Campylobacter* enteritis
   B   *Chlamydia trachomatis* infection
   C   Ischaemic colitis
   D   Radiation proctitis
   E   Ulcerative colitis

2. A 70-year-old man presents with an acute onset of severe generalised abdominal pain with few clinical signs. Routine blood tests show raised inflammatory markers.

   What is the most likely diagnosis?

   A   Acute mesenteric ischaemia
   B   Acute pancreatitis
   C   Diverticular disease
   D   Perforated duodenal ulcer
   E   Ruptured abdominal aortic aneurysm

3. A 33-year-old man presents with recurrent episodes of severe pain which is localised to the anus. The pain lasts for seconds and completely resolves in between attacks.

   What is the most appropriate management?

   A   Barium enema
   B   Colonoscopy
   C   CT of abdomen and pelvis
   D   Reassurance
   E   Topical glyceryl trinitrate 0.2%

4. Which of the following statements best describes hereditary non-polyposis colorectal cancer?

   A It accounts for 3–5% of all colorectal cancers
   B It can present with a Desmoid tumour
   C It is associated with Gardner's syndrome
   D It results in mutation of chromosome 5q21
   E Prophylactic colectomy and ileal pouch anal-anastomosis before age 20 years is recommended

5. A 14-year-old boy is diagnosed with familial adenomatous polyposis.

   Which is the most appropriate recommended management step?

   A Surveillance colonoscopy every 1–2 years from the age of 16 years onwards
   B Surveillance colonoscopy every 1–2 years from the age of 25 years onwards
   C Surveillance annual flexible sigmoidoscopy from age 13 years until age 30 years
   D Surveillance annual flexible sigmoidoscopy is recommended from age 30 years onwards
   E Upper gastrointestinal endoscopy from the age of 15 years

6. Treatment for mainstay of remission of ulcerative colitis includes aminosalicylates.

   Which of the following statements best describes aminosalicylates?

   A They are not available in topical preparations for treatment of colitis
   B 5-aminosalicylic acid (5-ASA) can lead to male infertility
   C 5-ASA is a purine analogue
   D Mesalazine products have been shown to increase the risk of colorectal cancer
   E Osteoporosis can occur in up to 50% of patients using aminosalicylates

7. Azathioprine and 6-mercaptopurine are used to maintain remission in ulcerative colitis and Crohn's disease.

   Which statement does not describe thiopurine therapy?

   A Purines affect folic acid synthesis and also DNA synthesis
   B It takes up to 6 weeks to show a clinical effect
   C Thiopurines are generally given orally based on a dose-weight regimen
   D Up to 66% of patients will respond to treatment with purines
   E Up to one-third of patients are intolerant, with nausea being the most common side effect

8. Following a diagnosis of acute fulminant colitis, a patient is commenced on cyclosporin.

   Which of the following statements best describes cyclosporine therapy?

   A Careful monitoring of serum drug concentration and renal function is required
   B It should be given as an oral preparation
   C It is given on an 8-weekly basis by intravenous infusion
   D It is the first licensed biological treatment
   E Treatment should only be given for 48 hours

9. A 64-year-old man presents with a small asymptomatic parastomal hernia 6 months after an abdominoperineal resection.

What is the next appropriate management step?

A   CT of the abdomen
B   Laparotomy and mesh repair of parastomal hernia
C   Laparotomy and resiting of stoma
D   Localised repair of parastomal hernia
E   Reassurance and stoma nurse input

10. An 82-year-old woman is reviewed at outpatient clinic complaining of a lump at her anus and faecal incontinence. Examination reveals concentric folds of mucosa protruding from her anus which can be manually reduced.

What is the most likely diagnosis?

A   Anal cancer
B   Circumferential skin tags
C   Full thickness rectal prolapse
D   Haemorrhoidal prolapse
E   Mucosal prolapse

11. A 64-year-old man is newly diagnosed with solitary rectal ulcer syndrome, having undergone flexible sigmoidoscopy and biopsies which confirmed the diagnosis.

What is the next appropriate management step?

A   Anterior resection
B   Biofeedback
C   Glyceryl trinitrate 0.2%
D   Local ulcer excision
E   Ventral rectopexy

12. A 40-year-old man presents with severe anal pain on defecation and fresh per rectal bleeding, which he only notices on the toilet paper. He is too sore to tolerate a per rectal examination at clinic.

What would be the most appropriate initial management?

A   50 U botulinum toxin injections locally to the anus
B   Anal dilatation
C   Colonoscopy
D   Lateral internal sphincterotomy
E   Glyceryl trinitrate (0.2–0.4%) applied topically

13. A 66-year-old woman undergoes adjuvant chemotherapy, following an anterior resection for Dukes stage C colonic cancer.

    Which of the following statements best describes adjuvant treatment of colorectal carcinoma?

    A Adjuvant treatment is started 1 year after surgery
    B Capecitabine is selectively converted to 5-fluorouracil (5-FU) by enzymes present in tumour cells
    C 5-FU is given alone
    D Oxaliplatin belongs to a family of drugs called antimetabolites
    E The decision for adjuvant treatment is taken by the surgeon alone

14. Which of the following is not a side effect of 5-fluorouracil?

    A Diarrhoea
    B Photophobia
    C Constipation
    D Dysgeusia
    E Palmar–plantar syndrome

15. A 65-year-old woman is diagnosed with an anal squamous cell cancer after an examination under anaesthesia and biopsies of an anal lesion.

    Which is the next most appropriate management step?

    A Anterior resection
    B 5-Fluorouracil and mitomycin C chemotherapy for 1 year
    C 5-Fluorouracil and mitomycin-C chemotherapy in combination with radical pelvic radiotherapy
    D Localised excision alone
    E Pelvic radiotherapy

16. Which of the following statements describes carcinoid of the colon and rectum?

    A Carcinoid usually occurs in the caecum
    B One-third of patients have nodal disease or distant spread at diagnosis
    C Surgery is not usually indicated
    D The median age at presentation is between 30 and 40 years old
    E Usual presentation is with carcinoid syndrome

17. Which of the following statements describes colonic lymphoma?

    A It accounts for 10% of all malignant large bowel neoplasms
    B It is more common in women
    C Hodgkin's lymphoma is the most common cause
    D Localised disease can be treated by surgical resection
    E The rectum is the most commonly affected site

18. A 68-year-old man with no past medical history undergoes polypectomy at 80 cm for a pedunculated polyp. Histopathological examination has shown invasive malignancy with carcinoma invading into the submucosa of the bowel wall but not through the muscularis propria. The site has been marked with Indian ink tattoo.

How would you proceed?

A   Colonic resection
B   Colonoscopic evaluation and repeat biopsy at 3 months
C   Transanal endoscopic microsurgery
D   Chemoradiotherapy
E   Colonoscopic surveillance 6 monthly

19. A 65-year-old man undergoes colonoscopy and is found to have a large sessile adenoma within the rectum which is removed piecemeal. The rest of the colon is normal. Histopathology confirms no invasive malignancy.

What is the most appropriate management?

A   3-monthly flexible sigmoidoscopy and re-examination of site
B   6-monthly colonoscopy
C   3-yearly colonoscopy
D   Annual colonoscopy
E   CT of abdomen and pelvis

20. A 72-year-old man undergoes colonoscopy for investigation of a change in his bowel habit. At colonoscopy two small polyps are removed from the sigmoid colon. The rest of the colon is normal. Histopathology subsequently confirms <1 cm adenomas.

What is the most appropriate management?

A   1-yearly colonoscopy
B   3-yearly colonoscopy
C   CT of abdomen and pelvis
D   No follow-up
E   Repeat colonoscopy in 2 months

21. A 68-year-old man is undergoing 3-yearly surveillance colonoscopy. He had three small adenomas excised in the past, one of which was greater than 1 cm. He has now had two consecutive negative examinations.

What is the most appropriate management?

A   Annual colonoscopy
B   Continue 3-yearly surveillance
C   No further surveillance
D   3-yearly barium enema
E   5-yearly colonoscopy

22. An 84-year-old woman with chronic obstructive pulmonary disease undergoes a successful colonoscopy and removal of four sessile polyps all <1 cm. Histopathology confirms them all to be adenomas.

What is the most appropriate management?

A   3-yearly colonoscopy
B   5-yearly colonoscopy
C   6-monthly colonoscopy
D   Annual colonoscopy
E   No further surveillance

23. A 23-year-old man has been diagnosed with an anal fissure, which has failed to heal with first line treatment.

What is the next most appropriate treatment?

A   5–10 units of botulinum toxin injected into the external sphincter
B   15–30 units of botulinum toxin injected into the external anal sphincter
C   15–30 units of botulinum toxin injected into the internal anal sphincter
D   45 units of botulinum toxin injected into the external anal sphincter
E   Prescription of 0.6% topical glyceryl trinitrate

24. A 24-year-old man is diagnosed with an intersphincteric fistula-in-ano during an examination under anaesthetic.

Which is the most appropriate treatment?

A   Biopsies of rectal mucosa only
B   Insertion of a 'cutting' seton
C   Insertion of a 'loose' seton
D   Laying open of the fistula
E   No surgical intervention and MRI of pelvis

25. A 33-year-old man presents with a perianal abscess at the 6 o'clock position.

Which of the following is the most appropriate management?

A   CT of the abdomen
B   Examination under anaesthetic and drainage of sepsis
C   Flexible sigmoidoscopy
D   Intravenous antibiotics
E   MRI of the pelvis

26. Which of the following statements best describes Crohn's disease (CD)?

A   >90% of patients with CD will require surgery
B   >90% of patients with ileocaecal CD will ultimately require resection
C   In 50% of cases of colitis it is not possible to differentiate between CD or ulcerative colitis (UC)
D   Oral ulceration is present is 15% of patients
E   The small intestine alone is involved in 80% of patients with CD

27. Which of the following statements best describes ulcerative colitis?

    A   Approximately 60% of patients present with proctitis
    B   Hypoalbuminaemia is only found in mild cases
    C   Pancolitis affects 40% of patients with ulcerative colitis
    D   The risk of colon cancer with pancolitis is 5% at 10 years
    E   The risk of colon cancer with pancolitis is 10% at 20 years

28. A 35-year-old man has severe acute ulcerative colitis which is not responding to maximal medical therapy. He is hypotensive and tachycardic with peritonitis.

What is the most appropriate treatment?

    A   Emergency panproctocolectomy only
    B   Emergency panproctocolectomy with ileo-pouch anal anastomosis
    C   Emergency subtotal colectomy and ileorectal anastomosis
    D   Emergency subtotal colectomy and ileostomy
    E   Increase dose of intravenous steroids

29. An 85-year-old woman presents with rectal prolapse. She is physically frail but mentally bright. Areas of the prolapsed rectal mucosa are necrotic.

What is the best treatment?

    A   Reduction of the prolapse, high fibre diet and stool softeners
    B   Anal encirclement procedure under local anaesthetic
    C   Resection rectopexy
    D   Perineal rectosigmoidectomy
    E   Sutured rectopexy

30. A newborn baby fails to pass meconium within 48 hours. A full thickness rectal biopsy is diagnostic of Hirschsprung's disease.

Which of the following are incorrect?

    A   Both the myenteric and submucosal plexuses are absent
    B   The RET protooncogene is implicated
    C   Hirschsprung's disease is most common in premature infants
    D   Hirschsprung's disease is associated with trisomy 21
    E   Hirschsprung's disease is associated with multiple neuroendocrine syndrome II

Questions: EMIs

Theme: Rectal bleeding

A   Anal cancer
B   Anal fissure
C   Diverticular disease
D   Fistula-in-ano
E   Haemorrhoids
F   Ischaemic colitis

G   Radiation proctitis
H   Rectal cancer
I   Rectal prolapse
J   Solitary rectal ulcer syndrome
K   Upper gastrointestinal source
L   Vascular malformation

Instructions: For each of the following scenarios, choose the single most likely diagnosis from the list above. Each option may be used once, more than once or not at all.

31. A 26-year-old man is investigated for rectal bleeding. A flexible sigmoidoscopy is undertaken and biopsies reveal that the lamina propria is replaced with smooth muscle and there is thickening and disruption of the muscularis propria.

32. A 40-year-old woman presents to the outpatient clinic with severe anal pain. Examination reveals a linear spilt in the mucosa of the anal canal.

33. A 28-year-old man presents with a recurrent perianal abscess. He undergoes incision and drainage of this, but it fails to heal and continues to discharge daily.

Theme: Infective diarrhoea

A   *Campylobacter*
B   *Clostridium difficile*
C   *Cryptosporidium hominis*
D   *Entamoeba histolytica*
E   *Escherichia coli*
F   *Giardia lamblia*

G   *Salmonella typhi*
H   Schistosomiasis
I   *Shigella dysenteriae*
J   *Strongyloides stercoralis*
K   Viral
L   *Yersinia enterocolitica*

Instructions: For each of the following descriptions, choose the single most likely infection from the list above. Each option may be used once, more than once or not at all.

34. A 79-year-old woman develops acute diarrhoea and is found to be Toxin A and B positive.

35. The most common cause of acute gastrointestinal infections.

36. An 18-year-old woman nursery nurse has developed symptoms including dermatitis, coughing, wheezing and abdominal pain.

Theme: Constipation

A   Amyloidosis
B   Anal stricture
C   Collagen vascular disease
D   Diverticular disease
E   Hirschsprung's disease
F   Inflammatory bowel disease

G   Irritable bowel disease
H   Megacolon (e.g. Chagas' disease)
I   Ogilvie's syndrome
J   Rectal prolapse
K   Scleroderma
L   Slow-transit constipation

Instructions: For each of the following descriptions, choose the single most likely diagnosis from the list above. Each option may be used once, more than once or not at all.

37. A 65-year-old woman has been in intensive care for 6 days with severe pneumonia. She has required invasive ventilation and haemofiltration. She develops abdominal distension. An abdominal X-ray reveals colonic distension with her caecum measuring 11 cm in diameter.

38. A 35-year-old man underwent open haemorrhoidectomy 1 year ago.

39. A 40-year-old woman presents with painful fingers and oesophageal reflux. Human leukocyte antigen gene mutation is present.

Theme: Polyposis syndromes

A   Desmoid tumour
B   Familial adenomatous polyposis
C   Gardner's syndrome
D   Hyperplastic polyposis
E   Juvenile polyposis
F   Lynch I

G   Lynch II
H   Muir–Torre syndrome
I   Osteomas
J   Peutz–Jeghers syndrome
K   Turcot's syndrome
L   Wegener's granuloma

Instructions: For each of the following scenarios, choose the single most likely diagnosis from the list above. Each option may be used once, more than once or not at all.

40. A 24-year-old woman is diagnosed with multiple colonic polyps after a colonoscopy, but is also noted to have skin lesions which include epidermoid cysts and keratoacanthoma.

41. A 13-year-old girl is found to have colonic polyps and is advised to have an annual flexible sigmoidoscopy.

42. A 12-year-old girl presents with multiple intestinal polyps and mucocutaneous pigmentation on her skin.

Theme: Bowel preparation

A   Fybogel (isphagula)
B   Glycerine
C   Loperamide (Imodium)
D   Klean-Prep
E   Lactulose
F   Magnesium citrate

G   None
H   Phosphate enema
I   Arachis oil enema
J   Senna (Senokot)
K   Sodium phosphate
L   Sodium picosulphate

Instructions: For each of the following descriptions, choose the single most likely treatment from the list above. Each option may be used once, more than once or not at all.

43. Improves the outcome of patients undergoing colorectal surgery.

44. A polyethylene glycol which, when made up to 4 L, can affect tolerability and compliance.

45. Can cause significant changes in electrolytes and should be avoided in patients with cardiac or renal problems.

Theme: Agents in the treatment of colorectal cancer

A   Capecitabine
B   Cetuximab
C   Corticosteroids
D   5-fluorouracil
E   Folinic acid
F   Gabapentin

G   Mitomycin C
H   Oxaliplatin
I   Radiofrequency ablation
J   Radiotherapy
K   Tegafur–uracil
L   Vascular endothelial growth factor

Instructions: For each of the following descriptions, choose the single most likely agent from the list above. Each option may be used once, more than once or not at all.

46. A 65-year-old man has been increasing pelvic pain from an advanced rectal cancer.

47. This is given along with a pyrimidine analogue to enhance its effect by inhibiting thymidylate synthase.

48. A 67-year-old man is receiving adjuvant treatment for a high-risk Dukes stage B adenocarcinoma and develops significant side effects of neutropenia and sensory neuropathy.

Theme: Anal fissure

A   Anal advancement flap
B   Anal dilatation
C   Onabotulinumtoxin A (Botox)
D   Calcium channel blocker
E   Diltiazem
F   Glyceryl trinitrate (GTN)
G   Hyperbaric oxygen therapy
H   Loperamide (Imodium)
I   Lateral internal sphincterotomy
J   Local excision
K   Nothing
L   Abdominoperineal resection

Instructions: For each of the following descriptions, choose the single most likely treatment from the list above. Each option may be used once, more than once or not at all.

49. A 33-year-old woman remains symptomatic from her fissure despite two courses of topical based therapies. She is recommended treatment which causes inhibition of acetylcholine at the neuromuscular junction by binding to presynaptic cholinergic nerve terminals.

50. Is as equally effective as the other topical therapy belonging to the calcium channel blocker drug group in the treatment of chronic anal fissure but is associated with higher rate of side effects.

51. A 66-year-old man has a chronic anal fissure and is being counselled that this course of treatment predisposes to incontinence of flatus and faecal soilage in up to 35% of patients.

Theme: Surveillance of colorectal conditions

A   Annual colonoscopy with 3-yearly upper gastrointestinal (GI) endoscopy
B   Annual colonoscopy ongoing
C   Annual colonoscopy until age 25 years
D   Annual flexible sigmoidoscopy
E   Biennial total colonic surveillance
F   3-yearly colonoscopy
G   3-yearly colonoscopy and upper GI endoscopy
H   3-yearly barium enema and sigmoidoscopy
I   5-yearly colonoscopy ongoing
J   5-yearly sigmoidoscopy ongoing
K   5-yearly colonoscopy until age 60 years
L   No surveillance recommended

Instructions: For each of the following descriptions, choose the single most likely surveillance from the list above. Each option may be used once, more than once or not at all.

52. A 25-year-old woman is newly diagnosed with hereditary non-polyposis colorectal cancer.

53. A 14-year-old boy who has been diagnosed with familial adenomatous polyposis.

54. A 16-year-old boy who has a strong family history of juvenile polyposis syndrome but is asymptomatic himself.

Theme: Inflammatory bowel disease treatment

A   Azathioprine
B   Cyclosporin
C   Ciprofloxacin and metronidazole
D   Hydrocortisone
E   Imodium
F   Infliximab
G   Observation only

H   Panproctocolectomy
I   Prednisolone
J   Subtotal colectomy and ileostomy
K   Subtotal colectomy and ileorectal
    anastomosis
L   Sulphasalazine

Instructions: For each of the following scenarios, choose the single most likely treatment from the list above. Each option may be used once, more than once or not at all.

55. A 28-year-old woman has had 5 days of intravenous steroid and monoclonal antibody therapy. Her bowel movements have decreased to 5 times per day, but she is now hypotensive and tachycardic.

56. A 44-year-old woman has an ileal pouch anal anastomosis and presents shortly after closure of ileostomy with frequency, urgency and liquid stool.

57. The first licensed biological treatment for Crohn's disease.

Theme: Anorectal pathophysiology

A   Anal fissure
B   Anal stenosis
C   Anismus
D   Carcinoma
E   Fistula-in-ano
F   Haemorrhoid

G   Internal rectal prolapse
H   Pruritus ani
I   Pudendal pain syndrome
J   Rectal sensory dysfunction
K   Rectocoele
L   Solitary rectal ulcer syndrome

Instructions: For each of the following scenarios, choose the single most likely diagnosis from the list above. Each option may be used once, more than once or not at all.

58. A 29-year-old woman presents to the outpatient clinic complaining of a burning sensation in the perineum which is constant. She reports that she needs to remain upright, as any pressure on the area when sitting exacerbates the pain. An MRI of her pelvis is normal.

59. A 56-year-old woman presents to clinic complaining of incompletely evacuating her rectum at defecation and having to digitate her vagina to defecate. A flexible sigmoidoscopy is normal, but she goes on to have a defecting proctogram which reveals prolapse of the rectum anteriorly.

60. A 60-year-old man has a defecting proctogram which shows a space-occupying lesion in the contrast filled rectum, despite a previously normal flexible sigmoidoscopy.

Answers: SBAs

1. D Radiation proctitis

This patient has the classical features and symptoms of radiation proctitis, commonly seen in men who have undergone radiotherapy for prostate cancer. This would be one of the common outpatient clinic referrals in such groups of patients. Patients may present with rectal bleeding and discharge, however with the nature of the underlying pathological process, strictures and sometimes fistulae can be identified. Anaemia would not be common with an infective cause and the history is very suggestive of a radiation proctitis rather than an inflammatory bowel disorder, although biopsies at the time of the flexible sigmoidoscopy may confirm the clinical suspicion.

2. A Acute mesenteric ischaemia

In this patient, it would be negligent for the surgeon to miss a diagnosis of acute mesenteric ischaemia as this is a classical presentation. Acute mesenteric ischaemia can present with vague clinical symptoms and mortality is high. Patients are usually elderly and present with severe abdominal pain but minimal clinical signs on examination, as in this scenario (unless of course a perforation of the bowel has occurred). An acidosis result on arterial blood gas should raise suspicions, as should an electrocardiogram finding of atrial fibrillation. Mesenteric angiography (or abdominal CT, if mesenteric venous thrombosis is suspected) remains the gold standard of diagnosis.

3. D Reassurance

Proctalgia fugax is characterised by, as in this case, sudden, severe attacks of anal pain without evidence of any anorectal conditions. These episodes of pain tend to self-resolve. A careful history and examination of the patient must be undertaken, including a per rectal examination. The patient may explain that attacks commonly occur at night and males more than females seem to be more affected. The cause of the pain remains unclear, but it has been thought that abnormal smooth muscle contractions may be an underlying factor. Between episodes of symptoms the patient is otherwise well. Reassurance is often all that is required, although patients may be referred for further investigations if there are any suspicions of an underlying anorectal pathology. In this case a flexible sigmoidoscopy or MRI of the pelvis may be appropriate. Topical glyceryl trinitrate (GTN) should only be prescribed if there is evidence of an anal fissure on examination or if the patient describes pain during or after defecation.

4. A It accounts for 3–5% of all colorectal cancers

Hereditary non-polyposis colorectal cancer (HNPCC) is a cause of 3–5% of colorectal cancers. It results from changes involving mismatch repair genes, unlike familial adenomatous polyposis (FAP) which affects chromosome 5q21 and is also associated with Gardner's syndrome and desmoid tumours. The average age at diagnosis of HNPCC is 45 years, with development of tumours in the proximal, rather than distal, colon and tumours are often multiple. Colonoscopy is recommended biennially from the age of 25 years onwards or 5 years younger than the age of diagnosis of the youngest affected individual. Therefore is important that all affected families are referred to a genetics team. The option of prophylactic colectomy can be discussed rather than surveillance, but there is as yet no data to recommend or dispute such surgery.

5. C Surveillance (with annual flexible sigmoidoscopy) from age 13 years until age 30 years

Patients with familial adenomatous polyposis should be advised to undergo prophylactic colectomy between the age of 16 years and 20 years to prevent development of a malignancy. However, until this is undertaken, surveillance of the large bowel is recommended in the form of yearly flexible sigmoidoscopy from 13–15 years of age and 5-yearly from 30–60 years of age. The undertaking of an upper gastrointestinal (GI) endoscopy from the age of 30 years is also advised because of the risk of upper GI polyps, which have malignant potential if they are not identified early.

6. B 5-aminosalycylic acid (5-ASA) can lead to male infertility

Aminosalicylates are available in topical form and are used for attempting to induce remission in ulcerative colitis and in the UK are licensed under various names such as Pentasa and Asacol. Sulphasalazine is a derivative of mesalazine. Up to 80% of men develop sperm dysmotility during treatment with aminosalicylates thus affecting their fertility; however, aminosalicylates have been shown to reduce the chances of developing colorectal cancer in patients who are prescribed them.

7. A Purines affect folic acid synthesis and also DNA synthesis

Azathioprine and 6-metacaptopurine (6-MP) are used to attempt to sustain a remission in inflammatory bowel disease. Thiopurines are purine analogues that affect multiple parts of the inflammatory cascade by affecting folic acid and DNA synthesis. It can take up to 6 weeks for a clinical response to manifest and over 30% of patients have side effects which cause them to stop taking the drug. Bone marrow suppression should be anticipated and monitored for in patients undergoing treatment with this family of drugs.

8. A Careful monitoring of serum drug concentration and renal function is required

In this patient, careful monitoring of renal function and serum toxicity levels are required as renal impairment is a common complication of cyclosporin use. Cyclosporin is used in the treatment of acute colitis in the hope of remission and in this indication for therapy; the drug is usually given intravenously, not orally. It should be started early if the patient has a poor response to steroids. It is a calcineurin inhibitor, preventing T-cell activation and is usually given for up to 7 days in the hope of achieving a clinical improvement.

9. E Reassurance and stoma nurse input

In patients suffering with parastomal hernias, only symptomatic hernias should be offered surgical treatment, although patients may insist upon operative repair, especially for large, unsightly hernias. In this example, the patient is only 6 months postinitial surgery and the hernia is small and asymptomatic. A CT is unlikely to change the management with regards to the hernia (but may be an option if surgery is to be undertaken). The patient should have been counselled preoperatively that parastomal hernias affect up to 60% of colostomies and 30% of ileostomies. Underlying conditions which increase the likelihood of developing this type of hernia include obesity, malnutrition, emergency surgery, constipation and poor surgical technique. Most parastomal hernias can be managed with input from good stoma care nurses advising on correct stoma bags and supportive garments, and this should be the first line management.

10. C Full thickness rectal prolapse

This is a classical description of a grade V rectal prolapse as there are concentric folds of mucosa prolapsing at the anus. No other pathology would account for this description. This can lead to a mechanical outlet obstruction as the prolapse obstructs the anal canal. Evacuation proctography identifies five grades of prolapse, however evidently a grade V prolapse can be diagnosed from the history and sometimes clinical examination if it is protruding.

- **Grade I** – descends no lower than the proximal limit of the rectocoele
- **Grade II** – descends into the rectocoele but not to top of anal canal
- **Grade III** – descends to top of anal canal
- **Grade IV** – descends into anal canal
- **Grade V** – protrudes from anus

Complete rectal prolapse can be a debilitating condition which causes faecal incontinence, especially in elderly, frail and usually female patients. A number of surgical options are now available, whether using a perineal approach such as the Delorme and Altemeier procedures, or via an abdominal approach. A Cochrane review (Bachoo et al., 2000) found that it was impossible to differentiate between the different surgical outcomes from procedures such as the Delorme procedure, laparoscopic rectopexy and laparoscopic resection rectopexy for prolapse, owing to poor sample sizes and weaknesses in the reported literature.

11. B Biofeedback

In this 64-year-old patient with solitary rectal ulcer syndrome (SRUS), first line management should be referral to a specialist physiotherapist for biofeedback which can lead to an improvement in symptoms in up to 75% of patients. Because SRUS is usually a result of straining, the patient must also be advised to avoid constipation with the use of regular laxatives. The stapled transanal rectal resection (STARR) procedure and ventral rectopexy are the mainstay surgical options when such a pathway is to be considered, if biofeedback and other conservative measures fail.

12. E Glyceryl trinitrate (0.2–0.4%) applied topically

Anal fissures are commonly seen in the colorectal clinic and this case illustrates a common presentation of anal fissure. Traditional surgical methods such as anal dilatation can lead to faecal continence by causing damage to the internal sphincter. First-line treatment for anal fissures is the use of glyceryl trinitrate (GTN) paste or diltiazem paste topically with success rates of 20–70%. It has been suggested that side effects associated with GTN (e.g. headaches) can reduce compliance, thus affecting success rates. A Cochrane review (Nelson et al., 2012) has found that in treating chronic anal fissures in adults, surgical procedures are more effective than all medical therapies but none of the medical therapies were associated with risk of incontinence.

13. B Capecitabine is selectively converted to 5-fluorouracil (5-FU) by enzymes present in tumour cells

Capecitabine is selectively converted to 5-FU by enzymes found in tumour cells. With regards to adjuvant therapy, recommendations are taken usually at a colorectal multidisciplinary team meeting as they can be complex and should be tailored to each individual patient and their comorbidities and pathological diagnosis. Most high-risk patients (Dukes stage B with extramural vascular invasion involvement and any lymph node involvement) will be given adjuvant treatment, which is combination therapy (not 5-FU alone) involving oxaliplatin/5-FU/folinic acid and duration of treatment is normally 6 months (not 1 year), if patients are deemed suitable for adjuvant therapy from a fitness viewpoint.

14. C Constipation

The side effects of 5-fluorouracil include diarrhoea, bruising, epistaxis, watery eyes, photophobia, metallic taste in mouth/alteration of taste (dysgeusia), nausea and vomiting, anorexia, anaemia, mouth ulcers, tiredness, palmar-plantar syndrome (redness of the soles of the hands and feet) and alopecia.

15. C 5-Fluorouracil and mitomycin-C chemotherapy are given in combination with radical pelvic radiotherapy

This patient should be discussed at a colorectal multidisciplinary team meeting prior to commencement of treatment. With regards to treatment of anal cancer, surgery no longer plays a central role in the treatment; instead, advances in survival with the use of mitomycin C and 5-FU in combination with pelvic radiotherapy remains the gold standard. If surgery were to be recommended, an abdominoperineal resection, not anterior resection, would be the operative procedure. Anal cancer is rare, with an incidence of 1:100,000 in the USA and between 230–300 new cases per year in England and Wales. Histopathology may reveal squamous, basaloid carcinomas or mucoepidermoid cancers.

16. A Carcinoid usually occurs in the caecum

Carcinoid of the large bowel usually arises in the caecum and the median age for presentation is between 50 and 70 years of age, not 30–40 years old. Rather than presenting clinically most carcinoids are found incidentally on colonoscopy whereas undergoing surveillance or investigation for another reason. Surgery remains the standard of treatment in non-metastatic carcinoid but two-thirds of patients with have distant disease at time of presentation, in which case symptom control becomes first line therapy. All patients should be discussed at a colorectal multi-disciplinary team meeting.

17. D Localised disease can be treated by surgical resection

Large bowel lymphoma is rare (0.2–0.4% of all large bowel malignancies) and there is a male, rather than female ascendancy, with a peak incidence occurring in the 5th–7th decades of life. Non-Hodgkin's lymphoma, rather than Hodgkin's lymphoma, is most common and the caecum, not rectum, is the most commonly diagnosed site. If it affects a particular site then surgical resection may be undertaken either for symptomatic reasons (i.e. strictures) or for diagnostic reasons (i.e. to allow tissue for to be obtained for pathological reasons).

18. A Colonic resection

The polyp in this 68-year-old man conforms to Haggitt Level 4 classification. Studies have shown that this requires formal surgical resection of the area affected, because of the increase in the risk of lymph nodes being affected outwith the bowel. Surgical resection allows proper treatment and staging should be carried out preoperatively along with discussion at the colorectal multidisciplinary team meeting, as for any other colorectal cancer. It is therefore important that when excising large polyps or polyps which are clinically suspicious, the site is marked with Indian ink staining at the time of endoscopic removal so that the site can be identified if further intervention or re-evaluation of the site is required in the future. The Haggitt classification is a histological classification of the extent of invasion of pedunculated malignant colorectal polyps (**Figure 3.1**).

Level 0 – This is not an invasive carcinoma and describes an in situ carcinoma or one which is intramucosal.

Level 1 – This is a malignancy which is confined to the polyp head and extending into the submucosa.

Level 2 – This describes a polyp cancer whereby the neck of the polyp has been infiltrated with carcinoma.

Level 3 – This is the classification if any level of the stalk of the polyp is involved.

Level 4 – This defines a carcinoma extending from the stalk and into the bowel wall.

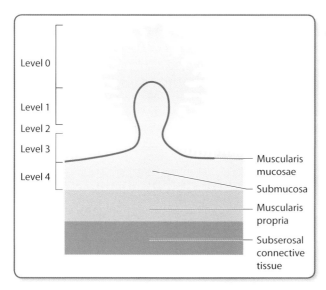

Figure 3.1 The Haggitt classification of pedunculated polyps.

19. A 3-monthly flexible sigmoidoscopy and re-examination of site

In this 65-year-old man, who has a piecemeal excision of a large sessile rectal adenoma, current guidelines (Atkins et al., 2002) suggest that follow-up should be a repeat endoscopy and re-look of the site of the adenoma excision 3 months after the initial excision. It is therefore imperative that the site is marked with Indian ink staining at initial colonoscopy. If the polyp has recurred and is not suitable for further endoscopic removal, then the patient should be assessed for surgical resection of the affected colon. However, if no further evidence of the polyp is seen on repeat endoscopy at 3 months, then a further examination should be undertaken at 1 year and then 3-yearly if appearances remain satisfactory.

20. D No follow-up

According to guidelines on adenoma removal by the British Gastroenterology Society and The Association of Coloproctology of Great Britain and Ireland (2002), there is no need to carry out further surveillance on this patient. He was found to have two small polyps at colonoscopy and they were both <1 cm, so he is in the low-risk category, which recommends no follow-up or 5-yearly follow-up until one negative examination.

21. C No further surveillance

The guidelines on adenoma removal (the British Gastroenterology Society and The Association of Coloproctology of Great Britain and Ireland; 2002) suggest that after two negative examinations no further follow-up is required. This patient had previously been categorised into the intermediate risk group and had undergone 3-yearly examinations and has now had two normal examinations. Follow-up can therefore be stopped.

22. E No further surveillance

This 84-year-patient has been found to be in the intermediate risk group with four small adenomas excised, all of which are <1 cm. The guidelines (the British Gastroenterology Society and The Association of Coloproctology of Great Britain and Ireland; 2002) for this group suggest that the patient should undergo 3-yearly examinations until two consecutive normal examinations. However, the patient is 84 years old and has chronic obstructive pulmonary disease, and the guidelines also suggest that surveillance can be stopped if the patient is >75 years of age or has significant comorbidities, which is the preferred pathway for this patient.

23. C 15–30 units of botulinum toxin injected into the internal anal sphincter

Anal fissures are commonly seen in the colorectal clinic. Traditional surgical methods such as anal dilatation are now outdated as they can lead to faecal incontinence by damaging the anal sphincter complex. When first-line treatment is medical, glyceryl trinitrate paste or diltiazem paste is applied topically; however, as in this case, up to 25% of patients fail to respond. The next appropriate step would be to perform an examination under anaesthesia and injection of 15–30 units botulinum toxin into the internal anal sphincter.

24. C Insertion of a 'loose' seton

This patient requires the insertion of a loose seton, rather than a cutting seton, to allow drainage of the sepsis. Fistulae-in-ano mostly arise as a result of anorectal sepsis but other conditions, such as Crohn's disease, can give rise to them and must be considered when patients with perianal sepsis are being assessed or treated. Biopsies should also be taken at the time of examination under anaesthesia (EUA) especially if there is a history of recurrent perianal sepsis or a family history of

Crohn's disease. If the fistula is low then imaging is not required, but clinically the surgeon must be certain that there is very limited or no sphincter involvement before laying open the fistula, because any damage to the sphincters could lead to faecal incontinence. A MRI should be arranged following examination under anaesthetic (EUA) and insertion of seton, to provide further clarification of the anatomy of the fistula – especially if it is thought to be complex (**Figure 3.2**).

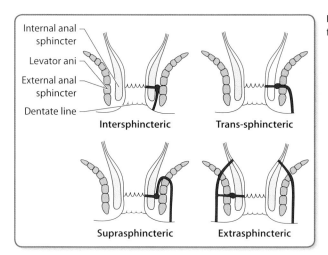

Figure 3.2 Park's classification of fistulous disease.

25. B Examination under anaesthetic and drainage of sepsis

In this patient, the most appropriate treatment would be examination under anaesthetic (EUA) and drainage of the underlying sepsis. Drainage should be carried out promptly to prevent the sepsis worsening. Perianal incisions to allow drainage of pus should be circumanal, thus reducing the likelihood of damage to the sphincters and thereby preventing faecal incontinence. However, if the patient presented with relatively little in the way of perianal symptoms but pelvic pain and pyrexia were the predominant symptoms, this may suggest a supralevator or pelvic abscess in which case an MRI of the pelvis may be the only way of diagnosing such patients. A CT of the abdomen and/or flexible sigmoidoscopy would add little to what information an EUA or MRI would provide and would not be the first choice. In patients with perianal sepsis it may be worth following up at outpatient clinic as 30% will have recurrent symptoms or an abscess that fails to heal because of the presence of a fistula-in-ano.

26. B >90% with ileocaecal CD will ultimately require resection

In >90% of patients with ileocaecal Crohn's disease (CD), surgery will be undertaken, mainly for strictures of the terminal ileum causing obstructive symptoms, or in some cases for histological diagnosis. CD cannot be discriminated from ulcerative colitis in 10–15% of cases of colitis, even in pathologically resected specimens. Thus management after emergency surgery can be difficult, especially if the patient has undergone a colectomy and end ileostomy as an emergency and wishes restorative surgery. If CD is the underlying diagnosis in this group of patients, then there is a high risk that any pouch surgery would fail.

27. D The risk of colon cancer with pancolitis is 5% at 10 years

The risk of developing colonic cancer in a patient diagnosed with pancolitis is 5% at 10 years and 20% at 20 years. 30%, not 60% of patients with ulcerative colitis (UC) present with proctitis and approximately 20%, not 40% of patients with UC have pancolitis. It is important that this group of patients is identified and surveillance is carried out, so that premalignant polyps can be identified and excised. A discussion between ongoing surveillance and formal surgical resection to avoid the risk of malignancy should also be undertaken with the patient. Hypoalbuminaemia is marker for disease severity and is a worrying indicator if present.

28. D Emergency subtotal colectomy and ileostomy

This 35-year-old patient has acute severe colitis with peritonitis. Toxic megacolon with perforation has a mortality rate of 30%. Patients with this diagnosis require urgent laparotomy and subtotal colectomy and ileostomy. As the patient is shocked, any anastomosis such as ileo-rectal or ileo-anal pouch or any prolonged procedure such as panproctocolectomy should not be undertaken. The patient should be fully resuscitated and given thromboprophylaxis and antibiotics preoperatively. A urinary catheter should also be in place. Peri- and postoperative immunosuppressants such as steroids should be closely monitored.

29. D Perineal rectosigmoidectomy

This patient has areas of mucosal necrosis and therefore cannot be managed conservatively unless a palliative pathway is chosen.

Anal encirclement is reserved for patients unfit for general anaesthesia. There is no difference in recurrence rates of prolapse between perineal and abdominal procedures and in a frail patient avoidance of an intra-abdominal approach may be more appropriate. If an abdominal procedure is carried out a minimally invasive approach may provide less morbidity and a reduced length of hospital stay.

30. C Hirschsprung's disease is most common in premature infants

Hirschsprung's disease is a congenital disorder occurring in 1:5000 live births. It is characterised by the absence of ganglia (both myenteric and submucosal plexuses) in the distal colon, resulting in a functional obstruction. Hirschsprung's disease occurs more commonly in males than females (4:1), and is uncommon in premature infants. It is associated with chromosomal abnormalities in approximately 9% of cases (such as Down's syndrome trisomy 21). Mutations in the RET protooncogene are associated with medullary thyroid cancer in MEN-2 and Hirschsprung's disease. Diagnosis is by full thickness rectal biopsies.

Answer: EMIs

31. J Solitary rectal ulcer syndrome

The early endoscopic findings in solitary rectal ulcer syndrome may only reveal patchy erythema of the mucosa such as in this patient. The characteristic histological findings are extension of the muscularis mucosa between crypts and muscularis propria disorganisation. Treatments such as biofeedback aim to return coordination to the pelvic floor, which can lead to symptom improvement. Surgery in the form of abdominal rectopexy may offer relief of symptoms in up to 50% of patients.

32. B Anal fissure

This 40-year-old patient has the symptoms and clinical findings of an anal fissure, which are commonly seen in the colorectal clinic. She should be advised of the reasons for a conservative approach to treatment in that traditional surgical methods such as anal stretch are now outdated, as they have been found to lead to faecal continence. If glyceryl trinitrate is the chosen therapy, she should be told that headaches are a common side effect. This affects compliance, in which case diltiazem paste may be the more appropriate treatment.

33. D Fistula-in-ano

This 28-year-old man has developed a fistula-in-ano, which must be suspected with his recurrent perianal sepsis. The reported rates of recurrent abscess or fistula development following simple incision and drainage of a perianal abscess range from 17% to nearly 90%. The most common classification system used to describe fistula-in-ano has been devised by Sir Alan Parks (**Figure 3.2**). In the presence of a recurring fistula-in-ano, the diagnosis of Crohn's disease must also be considered and ruled out and biopsies of rectal mucosa should be taken to allow this.

34. B *Clostridium difficile*

This patient has been diagnosed as having *Clostridium difficile* which is a Gram-positive, spore forming anaerobic bacillus. Diagnosis of *C. difficile* is by the presence of toxins A and B. 20% of antibiotic-associated diarrhoea is caused by this organism, although one-third patients with *C. difficile* infection have neither had a recent hospital stay, nor a recent course of antibiotics, which are the main factors for developing this infection.

35. K Viral

These are the most common infective source of acute gastrointestinal upset, with norovirus and rotavirus widespread. They are both common in the elderly and very contagious. If the diarrhoeal illness extends beyond 14 days it is described as 'persistent' diarrhoea. In a hospital setting, isolation of patients presenting with a diarrhoeal-type illness and stool cultures must be undertaken immediately, as well as rigorous implementation of infection control to stop the illness spreading.

36. J *Strongyloides stercoralis*

Strongyloides stercoralis is also known commonly as the threadworm and typically presents with symptoms including dermatitis, coughing, wheezing and abdominal pain, although up to 50% of carriers may be asymptomatic. The dermatitis is caused by penetration of the larvae through the skin, which can cause localised bruising. Pneumonia-like symptoms occur when the parasite has entered the lung cavity. Threadworms are common in children as they are often still learning good hygiene on visiting the toilet and it is easily spread.

37. I Ogilvie's syndrome

Ogilvie's syndrome is the acute dilatation of the colon in the absence of a mechanical obstruction, seen in critically unwell patients.

38. B Anal stricture

Anal stricture is a recognised complication of anorectal surgery. Mild stenoses may be managed with stool softeners or fibre supplements. Digital or manual dilatations may also be of benefit. Sphincterotomy may be utilised to surgically treat mild stenoses. In more severe cases anoplasty is required.

39. K Scleroderma

Scleroderma is an autoimmune condition associated with HLA gene mutation. Raynaud's phenomenon, caused by arterial spasm, is found in most patients at some point during their disease process. Systemic scleroderma, characterised by skin thickening due to accumulation of collagen, and small vessel vascular disease, involves not only the skin, hands, feet and face, but also the visceral organs. The gastrointestinal (GI) tract can be affected at any level with the most common symptom being oesophageal reflux, however GI dysmotility is also common and constipation (+/− alternating diarrhoea) can be problematic.

40. H Muir–Torre syndrome

This 24-year-old patient has a diagnosis of Muir–Torre syndrome which is described as a diagnosis of hereditary non-polyposis colorectal cancer (HNPCC) with associated skin lesions such as epitheliomas, epidermoid cysts, carcinoma and keratoacanthomas. It is an autosomal dominant condition.

41. B Familial adenomatous polyposis

Characterised by >100 adenomatous polyps of the colon and rectum, familial adenomatous polyposis (FAP) is an autosomal dominant syndrome and surveillance is recommended of the large bowel in the form of yearly flexible sigmoidoscopy from 13–15 years of age and 5-yearly from 30–60 years of age. Upper gastrointestinal endoscopy once patients reach aged 30 years is also recommended. The condition is due to mutations of the adenomatous polyposis coli gene on chromosome 5q.

42. J Peutz–Jeghers syndrome

This patient has multiple gastrointestinal polyps combined with mucocutaneous pigmentations, which are the underlying features of Peutz–Jeghers syndrome. Most individuals suffering from this autosomal dominant condition have a mutation in the serine/threonine kinase 11 (STK11) gene. The gastrointestinal polyps are hamartomatous polyps. Patients are not only at risk from developing gastrointestinal cancer, but also breast cancers. It is recognised that surveillance is important in the management of these patients to detect early or premalignant polyps but at present there are no defined guidelines.

43. G None

Güenaga et al. (2011) has looked at the effect of patient outcome if mechanical bowel preparation is used in colorectal surgery. It concluded that there is no benefit to the patient if mechanical bowel preparation is administered preoperatively. The review found that there was no difference in patient outcome, i.e. anastomotic leak rate, mortality or need for reoperation if bowel preparation was given or indeed avoided. It is felt that bowel preparation may be more disadvantageous to the patient by causing dehydration and electrolyte imbalance. However, if the patient is undergoing a full total mesorectal excision for a mid to low rectal cancer and a defunctioning ileostomy is to be given temporarily, then it may be that full bowel preparation will still be administered.

44. D Klean-Prep

Klean-Prep solution contains the active ingredient polyethylene glycol and is given orally in solution made up to 4 L. Although it has reported success rates of up to 90% in achieving a 'clean' colon and has little absorption properties, compliance is reduced by the volume required to ingest it.

45. K Sodium phosphate

Klean-Prep is given as a solution made up to 4 L, whereas sodium phosphate is taken in two 45 mL solutions. This may improve patient tolerance to sodium picosulphate but sodium phosphate solutions can lead to significant disturbances in serum electrolytes, in contrast to Klean-Prep solutions which cause minimal electrolyte disturbance.

46. J Radiotherapy

Radiotherapy can be used in both the neoadjuvant treatment of locally advanced rectal cancers to downstage them, and in the palliative setting to provide relief from bone metastases and pelvic pain in advanced cancers such as in this 65-year-old patient who has pelvic pain from advanced rectal cancer.

47. E Folinic acid

Folinic acid is used adjuvantly to enhance the effect of 5-fluorouracil in the adjuvant treatment of high-risk colorectal cancer patients, such as those with Dukes stage B carcinomas where there is extramural vascular invasion of the tumour or peritoneal involvement, or in lymph node positive patients (Dukes stage C) who are deemed fit enough to undergo chemotherapy.

48. H Oxaliplatin

The documented side effects of oxaliplatin use are neutropenia and sensory neuropathy. Oxaliplatin is given as adjuvant therapy for patients with high-risk colorectal cancer, as described in answer 47.

49. C Onabotulinumtoxin A (Botox)

This 33-year-old woman has had two courses of first line treatment with glyceryl trinitrate and diltiazem for her anal fissure, which has failed to respond, and she is now being recommended botulinum injections. Onabotulinumtoxin A reduces resting pressure and works by impairing the release of acetylcholine at the neuromuscular junction. 15–30 units of botulinum can be injected into the internal sphincter causing relaxation of the sphincter with reported healing rates of up to 70%. As the effects of this toxin wear off with time, the risks of faecal incontinence, as caused by surgical procedures such as internal sphincterotomy, are no longer present.

50. F Glyceryl trinitrate

With regards to the treatment of anal fissures, conservative treatment with both glyceryl trinitrate (GTN) and diltiazem paste have been shown to have similar success rates. GTN, however, is associated with an increased number of side effects such as headaches and anal pruritus which can obviously affect patient compliance.

51. I Lateral internal sphincterotomy

This patient is being counselled on the possible complications before embarking on a lateral internal sphincterotomy. Although studies in patients with anal fissures have shown that more favourable results may be gained through surgery, concerns still exist over the risk of causing faecal incontinence and conservative therapies are still preferred as first line treatments. Anorectal manometry should be carried out prior to any surgical procedure to assess sphincters – this is especially true in women who have undergone vaginal deliveries where sphincter damage may be present, thus increasing the risk of causing faecal incontinence further.

52. E Biennial total colonic surveillance

The guidelines for surveillance of patients with newly diagnosed hereditary non-polyposis colorectal cancer (Dunlop, 2002) suggest that 2-yearly, complete colonic surveillance, i.e. colonoscopy, is recommended from the age of 25 years (or 5 years less than the first diagnosed cancer in the family).

53. D Annual flexible sigmoidoscopy

In this case, the guidelines for patients diagnosed with familial adenomatous polyposis advise yearly flexible sigmoidoscopy from the ages of 13–15 years until the patient reaches the age of 30 (Dunlop, 2002). Once patients reach the age of 30 years, the guidelines advise that follow up should then be 3- to 5-yearly until the patient has reached their sixth decade of life.

54. B Annual colonoscopy ongoing

Here, large bowel surveillance for family members at risk of juvenile polyposis syndrome are recommended annually or biannually from the ages of 15–18 years or even earlier if the patient is symptomatic. Screening intervals could be prolonged once the age of 35 years old is reached.

55. J Subtotal colectomy and ileostomy

This patient is extremely unwell and needs an urgent laparotomy and subtotal colectomy and ileostomy. Medical management of her colitis has failed and she now has acute severe colitis. Although there are a number of classifications for acute colitis, Truelove and Witts provides a straightforward method of classification for such patients (see Table 1.2).

56. C Ciprofloxacin and metronidazole

This patient has a diagnosis of pouchitis which occurs early after closure of ileostomy. A first episode of pouchitis should be treated with ciprofloxacin and metronidazole.

57. F Infliximab

Infliximab is the trade name for the monoclonal antibody against tumour necrosis factor-α. Infliximab is used as the top tier treatment in the pyramid for medical management of inflammatory bowel disease and generally if patients do not respond to this treatment modality, surgery may be the next recommended step.

58. I Pudendal pain syndrome

This 29-year-old woman presents with symptoms typical of pudendal pain syndrome. This is pain perceived within the pelvis whereby no obvious injury or disease process is responsible, as in this patient who has undergone the normal MRI. It is a diagnosis of exclusion, much like irritable bowel disease. It is often extremely difficult to treat and patients must be reassured that no underlying malignancy is present. Often, as in this case, MRIs of the pelvis are usually normal and the treatment options are the same for any neuropathic conditions, with low-dose antidepressants useful.

59. K Rectocoele

This 56-year-old patient is presenting with the classical features of a rectocoele. This is a common problem with patients who present with the obstructive defecatory type symptoms of incontinence, digitating the vagina to assist defecation, pelvic pain and pelvic fullness. For diagnosis, an underlying malignancy must be excluded which may involve the patient being investigated with by a flexible sigmoidoscopy. A defecating proctogram can provide the diagnosis in patients with symptoms of a rectocoele, as the rectum prolapsing anteriorly into the vagina will be identified.

60. G Internal rectal prolapse

This 60-year-old patient has an internal rectal prolapse. He has no mass lesion within the bowel lumen until he strains on defecation. It is important to rule out a lesion within the rectum with a flexible sigmoidoscopy in the first instance. Internal rectal prolapse can present with symptoms of obstructive defecation and also faecal incontinence. Investigations of this include digital rectal examination to rule out a rectal lesion and flexible sigmoidoscopy may also be warranted to view the proximal rectum and distal sigmoid colon for prolapsing lesions. However, the gold standard investigation is a defecting proctogram. If any doubt remains then proceeding to Examination under anaesthetic should clarify the situation.

Chapter 4

Endocrine surgery

Questions: SBAs

For each question, select the single best answer from the five options listed.

1. A 60-year-old woman sustains a low impact fracture to her radius. She is found on dual-energy X-ray absorptiometry to have significantly reduced bone mineral density. Subsequently, her serum calcium is found to be raised at 2.9 mmol/L (2.2–2.6), with a parathyroid hormone level of 52 pmol/L (1.7–9.2). In the absence of renal disease, or other endocrine disorder, she has primary hyperparathyroidism. She is offered a targeted excision of a probable left inferior adenoma.

   What is the standard imaging required?

   A   Sestamibi scan and MRI, both consistent with a left-sided adenoma
   B   Sestamibi scan and ultrasound, both consistent with a left-sided adenoma
   C   Sestamibi scan with evidence of solitary adenoma on the left side
   D   Ultrasound and MRI, both consistent with a left-sided adenoma
   E   Ultrasound with evidence of solitary adenoma on the left side

2. A 24-year-old man presents to the outpatient department with an isolated, firm, midline swelling which has recently rapidly enlarged, becoming transiently painful. The patient thinks it is now regressing, measuring 1.5 cm. Fine-needle aspiration cytology of the lesion reveals only squamous debris.

   What is the most likely diagnosis?

   A   Reactive lymph node
   B   Sebaceous cyst
   C   Squamous cell carcinoma
   D   Thyroglossal cyst
   E   Thyroid cyst

3. A 70-year-old woman has undergone parathyroid surgery in a district general hospital for a suspected solitary right lower adenoma. The histopathology of the one resected lesion reveals only reactive lymph nodes. Her imaging, organised by the local endocrine surgical unit, is consistent on both sestamibi and ultrasound scan, for a left-sided adenoma.

   What operation is required?

   A   Formal neck exploration
   B   Targeted left-sided approach – endoscopic-assisted

    C Targeted left-sided approach – open
    D Targeted left-sided approach and proceed
    E Targeted right-sided approach – open

4. A 31-year-old woman has suffered from Graves' disease for 8 years and is increasingly troubled by thyroid eye disease. Her employment involves working with young children. She required hospitalisation for neutropenia during an earlier course of carbimazole, although she understands there are alternative drugs available. She wants to be treated again and her thyroid function is consistent with toxicity.

    What is the most appropriate treatment option?

    A Beta-blockade, then total thyroidectomy, pretreated with Lugol's iodine
    B Beta-blockade, then subtotal thyroidectomy, pretreated with Lugol's iodine
    C Propylthiouracil medication
    D Radiation therapy to her eyes
    E Radioiodine

5. A 40-year-old woman presents to thyroid outpatient clinic with tiredness, weight loss and heat intolerance; she has used lithium in the past for bipolar disease. She complains of a generalised neck swelling, and there is a family history of thyroid disease. On examination, she is clinically hyperthyroid, with lid lag and agitation. On examination, she has a smooth, palpable goitre with one dominant swelling (3 cm) in the right lobe.

    What is the most likely diagnosis?

    A Autoimmune thyroid disease
    B Colloid degeneration
    C Graves' disease
    D Lithium-induced thyroid disease
    E Toxic adenoma

6. A 65-year-old man is seen urgently at thyroid clinic with a rapidly growing neck swelling. He was previously fit and well, but for the last few weeks he has become weak, lost weight and is becoming short of breath when lying flat. On examination, there is an ill-defined, bilateral mass in the neck, causing a degree of tracheal deviation. He is uncomfortable bending forwards.

    What is the most appropriate treatment?

    A Chemotherapy
    B External beam radiation
    C Local debulking surgery
    D Palliative care
    E Radioiodine

7. A 60-year-old woman presents with a rapidly enlarging neck mass, associated with some dysphagia and voice change. She has no history of irradiation. Her general condition appears to be deteriorating fairly rapidly.

What is the most appropriate investigation?

A Core biopsy for histology
B Computed tomography
C Fine-needle aspiration cytology
D Ultrasound scan only
E Ultrasound scan and fine-needle aspiration cytology

8. A 34-year-old man presents with persistent hypertension, and on screening investigations, is found to have elevated urinary catecholamines consistent with phaeochromocytoma. This is subsequently confirmed on CT, which shows a 4 cm right-sided, well-defined, adrenal mass. The endocrinology team seek to control his blood pressure and sympathetic drive.

What is the most appropriate treatment?

A Bisoprolol
B Doxazosin
C Labetolol
D Metoprolol
E Phenoxybenzamine

9. What physiological abnormalities occur in primary aldosteronism (described by Conn)?

A Hypertension, elevated plasma renin activity and elevated aldosterone activity
B Hypertension, hypokalaemia and suppressed aldosterone activity
C Hypertension, suppressed plasma renin activity and elevated aldosterone activity
D Hypotension, elevated plasma renin activity and elevated aldosterone activity
E Hypotension, hyperkalaemia and elevated plasma renin activity

10. A 24-year-old woman presents with a cytologically-proven papillary thyroid cancer. She has a 2 cm intrathyroidal mass felt to the right of midline with neither palpable nodes, nor any nodes on ultrasound.

What is the most appropriate treatment?

A Right lobectomy and biopsy of any suspicious nodes
B Right lobectomy and central compartment nodal dissection
C Total thyroidectomy only
D Total thyroidectomy and central compartment nodal dissection only
E Total thyroidectomy, central compartment nodal dissection, clearance of right-sided III-VI nodes

11. A 60-year-old woman presents with primary hyperparathyroidism, and congruent imaging is consistent with a right superior parathyroid adenoma.

What is the embryological derivation of the superior parathyroid gland?

A The fourth pharyngeal pouch
B The second pharyngeal arch
C The third pharyngeal arch
D The third pharyngeal pouch
E The vestigial remnant of the ultimobranchial body

12. A 45-year-old woman is diagnosed with follicular thyroid cancer.

Which of the following pathological findings might you find?

A Parafollicular C cells
B Psammona bodies
C Hürthle cells
D Vesicular appearance of the nuclei of regional lymph nodes
E 'Orphan Annie-eye' nuclear inclusions

13. A 72-year-old woman is found to have an incidental 2 cm right-sided adrenal mass on a CT, which was performed for unexplained pain. She previously underwent treatment for locally advanced breast cancer 10 years ago, and is not known to be hypertensive.

What is the most appropriate investigation?

A Fasting cortisol and glucose
B Fine-needle aspiration of the lesion
C Repeat CT at 6 months
D Serial blood pressure recording
E Urinary catecholamine screen

14. A 45-year-old woman undergoes total thyroidectomy and central compartment dissection for a 5 cm papillary thyroid cancer, with biopsy-proven nodal disease. Her neck is cleared centrally, down to the mediastinum. The tumour had extrathyroidal spread laterally, and the recurrent laryngeal nerve (although visualised and exposed throughout its length) was closely adherent. In recovery, her cough and voice are abnormal and weak.

What is the most appropriate treatment?

A Analgesia
B Re-exploration of her neck
C Reintubation
D Saline nebulisers
E Tracheostomy insertion

15. A 56-year-old woman is seen at thyroid clinic and is being consented for a total thyroidectomy. Investigations have revealed a THY3 lesion (indeterminate on aspiration), dominant on the left, within a diffuse nodular thyroid. She is on no regular medications, and her baseline calcium is normal.

What are the procedural risks of complications?

A   0.2% risk of permanent recurrent laryngeal nerve injury, 10% risk of permanent hypocalcaemia

B   1% risk of haemorrhage and return to theatre, 5% risk of permanent hypocalcaemia

C   2% risk of haemorrhage and return to theatre, 0.1% risk of permanent recurrent laryngeal nerve injury

D   2% risk of permanent hypocalcaemia, 0.2% risk of permanent recurrent laryngeal nerve injury

E   5% risk of haemorrhage and return to theatre, 2% risk of permanent hypocalcaemia

16. A 48-year-old woman presents with a THY1 lesion (non-diagnostic on aspiration), aspirate from an isolated, recurrent 5 cm right-sided cystic thyroid swelling.

What is the most appropriate treatment?

A   Diagnostic lobectomy
B   Excision of cyst
C   Lobectomy and isthmusectomy
D   No operation
E   Total thyroidectomy

17. A 40-year-old woman has been noted to have a 4 cm papillary thyroid cancer (on cytology) in her right lobe, with no other palpable abnormality in her neck. Total thyroidectomy and right central compartment dissection is planned. She undergoes a preoperative ultrasound to complete her staging.

What finding on ultrasound would alter the management plan?

A   Multinodular disease throughout both lobes
B   No obvious nodal disease
C   Nodes (1 cm) at level IV on the right
D   Right thyroid mass without any ultrasound features of malignancy
E   Some lymph nodes <1 cm, with hypervascular signal, in the central compartment

18. A 60-year-old woman with hypercalcaemia, hyperparathyroidism, and osteoporosis undergoes a neck exploration in view of a lack of information in parathyroid imaging investigations. Her sestamibi scan failed to localise a lesion, and ultrasound was not helpful. The surgeon immediately finds a large, benign looking gland in the left inferior position, and a normal looking superior gland.

    What is the likelihood that the benign gland is the only pathological cause?

    A   <2%
    B   13%
    C   50%
    D   85%
    E   30%

19. A 12-year-old girl is seen at thyroid clinic with a strong family history of thyroid malignancy (medullary). She is a multiple endocrine neoplasia-2A kindred, with relatives diagnosed in their early twenties.

    What is the most appropriate serum marker to gauge the extent of disease?

    A   Carcinoembryonic antigen
    B   Serum calcitonin
    C   Serum chromogranin
    D   Serum free calcium levels
    E   Serum thyroglobulin

20. A 58-year-old woman undergoes an abdominal CT during investigations for bowel symptoms. The scan is reported as showing 'a 5 cm heterogeneous lesion in the right adrenal gland'. She is entirely asymptomatic from any possible functional lesion.

    What determines the malignant potential of this lesion?

    A   Age of the patient
    B   Family history of endocrine disorders
    C   Functional results from urinary metanephrine/normetanephrine collections
    D   Sex of the patient
    E   Size of the lesion

21. A 46-year-old man undergoes an abdominal CT for persistent, unexplained abdominal pain and is found to have a 3.5 cm left-sided adrenal mass. He has no documented history of hypertension, and remains well, on no regular medication.

    What statement best describes adrenal lesions?

    A   50% of phaeochromocytomas are diagnosed from incidentalomas
    B   Resection of the lesion is likely to resolve his pain
    C   Resection should be offered immediately
    D   There is a 10% risk this lesion is malignant
    E   There is a 5% chance that this lesion is a phaeochromocytoma

22. A 38-year-old man presents to thyroid clinic with a left-sided neck swelling. He is otherwise fit and well. On examination, he has a hard, 4 cm nodule palpable within his left thyroid lobe, and no obvious lymphadenopathy.

What is the most appropriate investigation?

   A   Fine-needle aspiration cytology (FNAC) and CT
   B   Freehand FNAC of the thyroid and chest X-ray
   C   Thyroglobulin estimation, ultrasound and biopsy
   D   Thyroid function and CT
   E   Ultrasound scan, FNAC of thyroid and nodal scan

Questions: EMIs

Theme: Tumours associated with genetic conditions

A   Adrenocortical carcinoma
B   Follicular carcinoma of the thyroid
C   Hepatoblastoma
D   Medullary carcinoma of the thyroid
E   Anaplastic cancer of the thyroid
F   Pancreatic neuroendocrine tumours
G   Papillary carcinoma of the thyroid
H   Parathyroid adenoma
I   Phaeochromocytoma

Instructions: For each of the following genetic disorders, choose the single most likely tumour from the list above. Each option may be used once, more than once or not at all.

23. A 26-year-old woman, whose mother had breast carcinoma and osteosarcoma, is found to carry a germ-line mutation in the p53 tumour suppressor gene, consistent with Li–Fraumeni syndrome.

24. A 38-year-old man presents with features of weight gain and lethargy, and is eventually diagnosed with an insulinoma; he has a genetic mutation consistent with multiple endocrine neoplasia-1. He is then screened for the other most commonly associated tumour.

25. A 4-year-old infant is referred to the endocrine surgical department for total thyroidectomy. His father was recently found to have a form of thyroid carcinoma and required extensive neck dissection to clear the disease. Genetic testing has been undertaken and confirms *RET* (the REarranged in Transfection proto-oncogene, a tyrosine kinase receptor gene) mutation.

Theme: Pathological diagnosis of endocrine tumours

A   C-cell hyperplasia
B   Chromogranin A stain positive
C   Lymphovascular invasion
D   None of these options
E   Orphan Annie eyes
F   THY5 (consistent with malignancy) on fine-needle aspiration cytology
G   Tumour capsular breach
H   Tumour deposits with lymph nodes resected at surgery
I   Weiss criteria

Instructions: For each of the following scenarios, choose the single most likely pathological feature for determining management from the list above. Each option may be used once, more than once or not at all.

26. A 34-year-old woman presents to the outpatient department with a hard, suspicious 3 cm nodule arising from her right thyroid lobe. She has enlarged lymph nodes along the jugular chain.

27. A 61-year-old man undergoes laparoscopic resection of a 4 cm adrenal lesion, with a preoperative diagnosis of phaeochromocytoma based on urinary collection of catecholamines. The decision on treatment will be determined by the presence of malignancy and metastases.

28. A 50-year-old woman undergoes total thyroidectomy for a 3 cm nodule in the left lobe. Preoperative fine-needle aspiration cytology is reported as consistent with medullary carcinoma. There is no family history and genetic screening is negative.

Theme: Thyroid goitre

A   Anaplastic carcinoma
B   Chronic lymphocytic thyroiditis
       (Hashimoto's disease)
C   de Quervain's thyroiditis
D   Diffuse goitre of pregnancy

E   Graves' disease
F   Multinodular goitre
G   Retrosternal goitre
H   Riedel's thyroiditis
I   Tuberculous thyroiditis

Instructions: For each of the following scenarios, choose the single most likely diagnosis from the list above. Each option may be used once, more than once or not at all.

29. A 40-year-old woman presents to thyroid clinic with a history of long-standing, slowly enlarging neck swelling. Her thyroid-stimulating hormone level is elevated and her thyroid autoantibodies positive. She has a family history of thyroid disease.

30. A 32-year-old man presents to his GP. He has had a flu-like illness for 1 week, with upper respiratory symptoms, and has since developed a diffusely tender swelling in his neck, with some odynophagia.

31. A 60-year-old woman presents with rapid onset swelling in her neck. She is otherwise well, but complains of some choking and dysphagia. Examination reveals a hard, fixed diffuse swelling of a small thyroid gland.

Theme: Thyroid cancer

A   Debulking surgery then external beam
       radiation therapy
B   External beam radiation therapy
C   Lobectomy alone then
       thyroid-stimulating hormone (TSH)
       suppression
D   Radioiodine treatment following
       appropriate surgery to the neck
E   Systemic chemotherapy

F   Total thyroidectomy and central node
       dissection
G   Total thyroidectomy and lateral node
       dissection (selective neck dissection)
H   Total thyroidectomy then TSH
       suppression
I   Total thyroidectomy, central node
       dissection, and lateral node dissection
       (selective neck dissection)

Instructions: For each of the following scenarios, choose the single most likely treatment from the list above. Each option may be used once, more than once or not at all.

32. A 23-year-old woman presents to the surgical outpatient department with an isolated 1 cm swelling of her right thyroid lobe. Ultrasound assessment and fine-needle aspiration cytology (FNAC) are carried out, which demonstrate a solitary, calcified 0.8 cm lesion, and cytology is reported as 'suspicious'. The thyroid is otherwise normal and no lymph nodes are reported as abnormal on the scan.

33. A 62-year-old man presents to the orthopaedic trauma unit with a fracture to his right hip. On investigations, this is found to be a pathological fracture, and his serum thyroglobulin is found to be >1000 µg/L. A bone scan reveals further 'hot spots' in his ribs and his chest radiograph is suspicious of metastatic disease. His hip is pinned successfully.

34. A 79-year-old woman presents as an emergency with stridor to the ear, nose and throat ward, having been complaining of a rapidly growing swelling in her neck over the previous 6 weeks. Palpation reveals a hard, irregular swelling measuring over 10 cm, and her voice is hoarse.

Theme: Adrenal tumours

A   CT-guided biopsy
B   Dexamethasone suppression test
C   Laparoscopic excision biopsy
D   Open excision biopsy
E   PET-CT

F   Repeat CT scanning at annual interval(s)
G   Serum renin:aldosterone ratio
H   Urinary and serum cortisol levels
I   Urinary catecholamine collection

Instructions: For each of the following scenarios, choose the single most likely investigation from the list above. Each option may be used once, more than once or not at all.

35. A 45-year-old woman presents with intermittent abdominal pains, most likely attributable to gallstones. Because of atypical features and a family history of pancreatic cancer, she undergoes a CT. This reveals a 2 cm lesion in her left adrenal gland 'in keeping with a myolipoma'.

36. A 70-year-old woman, previously treated 8 years ago for breast cancer, undergoes a CT of her abdomen and pelvis, arranged by her gynaecologist. No pelvic pathology is seen but a 4 cm heterogeneous lesion is reported on the right adrenal gland.

37. A 47-year-old man has been attending medical outpatients for 2 years with persistent hypertension which has not adequately responded to standard therapy. His serum cortisol is found to be marginally elevated and a CT of his abdomen reveals bilateral hyperplastic adrenal glands.

Theme: Parathyroid diagnoses

A   Four-gland parathyroid hyperplasia
B   Hyperparathyroidism jaw-tumour syndrome
C   Multiple endocrine neoplasia-1 (MEN-1) syndrome
D   Multiple endocrine neoplasia-2A (MEN-2A) syndrome

E   Multiple endocrine neoplasia-2B (MEN-2B) syndrome
F   Pleomorphic adenoma
G   Primary hyperparathyroidism
H   Secondary hyperparathyroidism
I   Tertiary hyperparathyroidism

Instructions: For each of the following scenarios, choose the single most likely diagnosis from the list above. Each option may be used once, more than once or not at all.

38. A 48-year-old woman had established renal failure secondary to diabetic nephropathy, for 10 years, until 1 year ago when she underwent a successful renal transplant. She now presents to acute medical services with painful white lesions on her shins and forearms, and is found to have a serum calcium level of 3.1 mmol/L.

39. A 57-year-old woman presents to the emergency department with a Colles' fracture which she sustained with minimal trauma. She undergoes routine dual-energy X-ray absorptiometry scanning, which reveals significantly reduced bone mineral density scores. Her serum calcium is found to be elevated at 2.91 mmol/L, with a parathyroid hormone level of 32 pg/mL.

40. A 26-year-old woman presents with weight loss and is found to have elevated serum glucose. She is presumed to have type 1 diabetes. On further investigation, her serum calcium is found to be elevated at 2.86 mmol/L, with a parathyroid hormone of 41 pg/mL.

Theme: MEN syndromes

A	Adrenocortical carcinoma	F	Midgut carcinoid tumour
B	Conn's adenoma	G	Pancreatic carcinoma
C	Gastrinoma	H	Parathyroid carcinoma
D	Glugagonoma	I	Phaeochromocytoma
E	Insulinoma		

Instructions: For each of the following scenarios, choose the single most likely diagnosis from the list above. Each option may be used once, more than once or not at all.

41. A 32-year-old man with hypertension has been found to have hypercalcaemia secondary to primary hyperparathyroidism. There is no family history of this disease, and his parathyroid imaging is consistent with four-gland hyperplasia. Abdominal scanning has picked-up a mass requiring further investigations.

42. A 24-year-old woman, whose father had pancreatic and parathyroid surgeries, presents with a perforated duodenal ulcer on a background of long-standing proton pump inhibitor use. She is found to be hypercalcaemic with elevated parathyroid hormone.

43. A 30-year-old man with MEN-1, previously having undergone total parathyroidectomy, presents with weight gain and lethargy.

Theme: Swellings in the neck

A	Chemodectoma	F	Metastatic squamous cell carcinoma
B	Cystic hygroma	G	Multinodular goitre
C	Globus hystericus	H	Pharyngeal pouch
D	Lymphoma	I	Solitary toxic nodule
E	Metastatic papillary carcinoma	J	Thyroglossal cyst

Instructions: For each of the following scenarios, choose the single most likely diagnosis from the list above. Each option may be used once, more than once or not at all.

44. A 17-year-old man presents to the outpatient clinic with a slightly tender, erythematous nodule in his neck, palpable just to the left of midline and which moves on swallowing, and on protrusion of the tongue.

45. A 70-year-old woman, previously treated with anxiolytics, presents to surgical outpatients with a 'feeling of something stuck in her throat' and thinks there may be a lump in her neck. She has had some difficulty swallowing, and her husband reports that she sometimes brings up partly chewed food with minimal effort. There is no palpable abnormality in her neck.

46. A 35-year-old-woman, who has smoked for 15 years, presents complaining of swelling in her neck. She has palpable lymphadenopathy in the right internal jugular chain, and posterior triangle. In addition, she has a 2 cm, hard swelling to the right of the midline which moves on swallowing.

Theme: Biochemical markers of neuroendocrine disease

A   5-Hydroxyindoleacetic acid level
B   Calcitonin
C   Chromogranin
D   Gastrin
E   Insulin/glucose
F   Renin:aldosterone ratio
G   Somatostatin
H   Thyroglobulin
I   Vanillylmandelic acid level

Instructions: For each of the following scenarios, choose the single most likely test from the list above. Each option may be used once, more than once or not at all.

47. A 35-year-old man presents with abdominal pain, diarrhoea and flushing.

48. A 33-year-old woman presents with upper abdominal pain and diarrhoea. She has previously been treated for renal stones. She has a history of multiple cancers in the family.

49. A 45-year-old man has been seeing his GP with headaches, weight loss and sweating. His blood pressure is recorded as 220/120 mmHg.

Theme: Parathyroid strategies

A Cinacalcet treatment
B Endoscopic-assisted total
   parathyroidectomy
C Formal subtotal parathyroidectomy
D Formal total parathyroidectomy
E No treatment, discharge

F No treatment, review in a year
G Parathyroid exploration, biopsy all
   glands
H Parathyroid exploration, remove
   abnormal glands
I Targeted excision of one gland

Instructions: For each of the following scenarios, choose the single most likely treatment from the list above. Each option may be used once, more than once or not at all.

50. A 78-year-old man with dialysis-dependent renal failure and comorbid cardiorespiratory disease has increasing metabolic problems with phosphate and calcium levels. He has intermittent headaches and suffers constipation. He is also found to have an elevated parathyroid hormone at 34 pmol/L. A sestamibi scan is suggestive of four-gland hyperplasia which is presumed secondary hyperparathyroidism.

51. A 50-year-old woman with a strong family history of osteoporosis arranges to undergo a 'well woman' check around the time of her menopause. This reveals that her serum calcium is elevated at 2.78 mmol/L, and her parathyroid hormone is also raised. With the suspicion of primary hyperparathyroidism, she undergoes sestamibi and ultrasound scans of her neck, which reveal concordant images suggestive of a left inferior parathyroid gland adenoma. She is keen to avoid a significant scar.

52. A 76-year-old man is admitted to hospital with a myocardial infarction from which he makes a good recovery and returns to a normal quality of life. Six weeks later, his GP explains that 'routine' clinical blood tests during his admission have revealed a calcium level of 2.7 mmol/L. The patient remains entirely asymptomatic, but he has a slightly elevated parathyroid hormone at 11 pg/mL, and discordant imaging. He is not keen for any further medical attention for now.

Answers: SBAs

1. B Sestamibi and ultrasound, both consistent with a left-sided adenoma

In primary hyperparathyroidism from a solitary adenoma, the minimum accepted imaging for a parathyroid exploration is a sestamibi scan. Scintigraphy provides sensitive and specific imaging. However, if the patient wishes a targeted approach (either limited incision, open surgery, or endoscopic assisted), the minimum accepted imaging is a combination of ultrasound and sestamibi (see **Table 4.1** for combined sensitivities). Axial imaging should only be necessary for second line surgery after a failed operation.

In **Table 4.1**, the approximate combined sensitivities and specificities of the varying forms of parathyroid imaging techniques are shown. Particularly in the reoperative setting, there is now a tendency to combine the functional information from the sestamibi scan with axial imaging in the form of a single-photon emission computed tomography scan; this is replacing the more invasive angiography and sampling, which were previously deemed to be gold standard in reoperations.

Table 4.1 Investigations to identify parathyroid adenomas		
Study	Sensitivity (%)	Specificity (%)
Ultrasound	75	80
CT with intravenous contrast	65	80
Sestamibi scan	91	99
Angiogram with venous sampling	–	97

2. D Thyroglossal cyst

This patient has a thyroglossal cyst. He is a young man, and these lesions may present within the first few decades of life. They only become obvious if an event, such as a small bleed into the cyst, occurs (as in this patient's case). Fine-needle aspiration cytology typically yields squamous cells. It can occur at several levels (**Figure 4.1**) although the position of the cyst in the midline is diagnostic, rising on protrusion of the tongue. Relations of the thyroid in the neck illustrate the descent of the gland from the foramen cecum at the base of the tongue. This explains why persistence of this track may predispose to thyroglossal cyst formation, with squamous lining. The ongoing attachment of the cyst to the foramen cecum creates the upward movement seen on protrusion of the tongue.

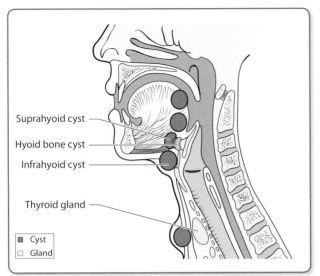

Figure 4.1 Anatomical sites of thyroglossal cysts.

Suprahyoid cyst

Hyoid bone cyst

Infrahyoid cyst

Thyroid gland

■ Cyst
□ Gland

3. D Targeted left-sided approach and proceed

This scenario represents revisional parathyroid surgery. In the absence of adequate imaging in the first presentation, it is reasonable to view the situation as a primary approach, within expert hands. Thus, with consistent dual imaging at 99% combined sensitivity for a left-sided lesion, despite earlier events, it is reasonable to offer targeted surgery. This may be open or endoscopic, depending on local expertise, but with a low threshold for proceeding to formal exploration should the adenoma not be found. A stepwise approach to investigating the various likely positions should be utilised, with the end point being a thyroid lobectomy on that side (**Table 4.2**).

Table 4.2 Suggested operative schema for localising parathyroid adenoma, in progressive order of 'invasiveness' or complexity, and decreasing likelihood	
Superior gland	In fat pad on thyroid surface, caudal to inferior thyroid artery
	Inferiorly, behind the inferior thyroid artery and oesophagus
	Behind the upper pole – divide superior thyroid pedicle and rotate upper pole anteriorly
Inferior gland	Along the thyrothymic axis
	Under capsule of lower pole of thyroid
	Down to accessible mediastinal thymus
	Within the carotid sheath
	Intrathymic – perform transcervical thymectomy
	Within thyroid lobe – may require thyroid lobectomy

4. A Beta-blockade, then total thyroidectomy, pretreated with Lugol's iodine

The risk of re-treatment in the context of previous agranulocytosis is too high and cannot be advocated. Although radioiodine could be given, in a young woman still of child bearing potential, who works with young children, this approach is not ideal. Although thyroid eye disease may eventually require external beam treatment, regression is possible with further management (this would not be advocated now). Instead, this patient should be offered total thyroidectomy, with control of toxicity with beta-blockade. There was a transient fashion for subtotal resection, but rates of recurrence and difficult revisional surgery have made this unattractive. This is particularly the case as this patient was unlikely to avoid thyroxine replacement therapy anyway.

5. E Toxic adenoma

Given the clinical picture of hyperthyroidism and the findings in the neck, toxic adenoma is the most likely diagnosis. Although Graves' disease is more common, this patient is too old for her first presentation. Lithium therapy is associated with: (i) the need to monitor thyroid function, and (ii) the development of thyroid swelling (both generalised and nodular, which may regress).

6. B External beam radiation

The differential diagnosis here is between anaplastic thyroid cancer and lymphoma. However, this patient also has symptoms of superior vena caval obstruction. This represents an oncological emergency, and a radiation oncologist should be asked to arrange appropriate treatment urgently. The patient will require admission with appropriate airway precautions available (as there is a danger of transient increased swelling). A core biopsy is also urgently required because, if a lymphoma is confirmed, chemotherapy may then be curative. Anaplastic cancer is unlikely to respond to neither chemotherapy nor radioiodine, and given the terrible

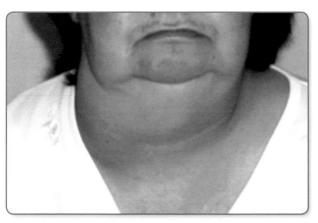

Figure 4.2 Anaplastic thyroid cancer. Locally advanced, aggressive anaplastic carcinoma, presenting as a rapidly enlarging, obstructive neck swelling in an older patient.

prognosis, debulking surgery may not be appropriate at this stage. Surgery is only recommended when the disease is limited to the thyroid/strap muscles, such as case illustrated in **Figure 4.2**.

7. A Core biopsy for histology

In a patient with this presentation, the differential diagnosis is between lymphoma and anaplastic carcinoma of thyroid. The former carries a grim prognosis and essentially needs rapid palliative care, with no reliable treatment modalities defined. Lymphoma, however, will respond well to systemic therapy and irradiation. Therefore, differentiation between these is crucial, and histology is required as cytology may be unreliable. The other investigations are useful in the work-up of a locally extensive, differentiated thyroid cancer. For reviews of the challenges faced in the rarer form of thyroid malignancy refer to Ain (1999) and Austin et al., (1996).

8. E Phenoxybenzamine

This is the preferred α-blockade regime, by which patients are loaded with the drug until some side effects are present, the most reliable of which is nasal congestion. Although beta-blockade may be required around the perioperative period, if the patient remains tachycardic, this is of secondary concern in the management of the systemic vasculature. Because of the vascular dilatation and effects of surgery, patients may then have large volume fluid requirements around surgery. Invasive monitoring will be required with a minimum of a central venous line and arterial line. Doxazosin may be used as an alternative in patients intolerant of phenoxybenzamine. O'Riordan (1997) provides a simple physiological summary.

9. C Hypertension, suppressed plasma renin activity and elevated aldosterone activity

Conn's syndrome is characterised by hypertension, with hyperaldosteronism leading to negative feedback on the renin axis (**Figure 4.3**). Conn's syndrome is also associated with hypokalaemia, through increased urinary losses of potassium. Increasingly, the plasma aldosterone:renin ratio is being used as a diagnostic test. This has resulted in the estimated prevalence of Conn's syndrome among hypertensive patients rising from 1.5% to ≥8%. The most common cause is bilateral idiopathic hyperaldosteronism.

The complex, multiorgan involvement in the renin–aldosterone hormone axis is illustrated in **Figure 4.3**, whereby the mechanism for the hypertension and metabolic disturbance may be fully understood.

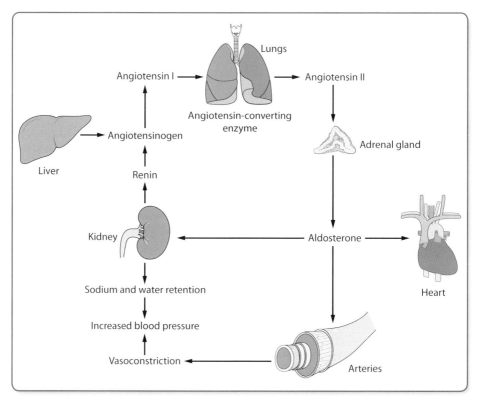

Figure 4.3 The renin–aldosterone axis.

10. D Total thyroidectomy and central compartment nodal dissection only

This patient, by age alone, has low-risk disease, and the consensus now is that unless there is proven nodal disease preoperatively, the extent of nodal dissection should be limited to diagnostic central compartment dissection (British Thyroid Association Guidelines, 2014). In addition, it is now accepted practice that total thyroidectomy is performed for all tumours >1 cm at first surgery. A 'cherry-picking' approach is not advocated. If suspicious nodes are found intraoperatively, this should be confirmed on frozen section, and a compartment-orientated dissection carried out if positive.

11. A The fourth pharyngeal pouch

The parathyroid glands derive from the pharyngeal pouches. The superior parathyroid glands are derived from the fourth and the inferior from the third pouch. The descent of the inferior parathyroid glands is longer than the superior parathyroid glands and is intimately associated with the development of the thymus. Hence there is more variation in the final position of the inferior parathyroid glands. Their embryological origins are illustrated in **Figure 4.4**. Approximately

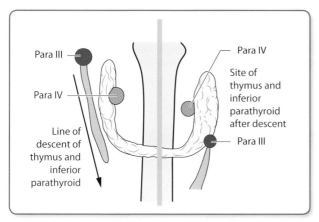

Figure 4.4 Parathyroid embryology. The longer path of descent of the inferior gland, derived from the third pouch (III), explains how their eventual location is more variable than that of the superior gland, which is derived from the fourth pouch.

50% of inferior parathyroid glands are located near the inferior pole of the thyroid gland and 30% in the thyrothymic ligament. A key paper by Thompson et al. (1982) provides an excellent overview.

12. C Hürthle cells

Hürthle cell carcinoma is considered a variant of follicular cell thyroid cancer. In contrast:

- Parafollicular C cells of neural crest origin are seen in medullary thyroid cancer
- Psammona bodies and 'Orphan Annie-eye' nuclear inclusions are seen in papillary thyroid cancer
- Vesicular appearance of the nuclei of regional lymph nodes is seen in anaplastic thyroid carcinoma with regional lymphadenopathy

13. B Fine-needle aspiration of the lesion

In the case of any adrenal mass, a phaeochromocytoma must be excluded, however in this case, we know the patient is not hypertensive. Exclusion of functional tumours requires serial blood pressure recordings, urinary catecholamine screen and fasting cortisol and glucose. These tests are all the more urgent if there is a firm indication for surgery, i.e. the mass is >4 cm. In the context of an incidental adrenal mass, the same size criteria, or rapid enlargement on serial scanning, apply. Given the history of cancer and the relative lack of indication for surgery, fine-needle aspiration of the lesion is required as a diagnosis of exclusion.

With increased use of axial imaging, including scanning of the 'worried well', there has been a significant increase in the reporting of incidental adrenal lesions by radiologists. For such lesions, like the one seen in **Figure 4.5**, a clear protocol must be in place to ensure over-investigation does not result in harm.

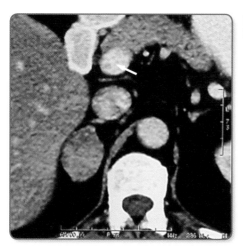

Figure 4.5 High-power CT of adrenal incidentaloma (arrowed).

14. D Saline nebulisers

This situation probably represents a transient palsy of the recurrent laryngeal nerve because of bruising and ischaemia during the procedure. If the nerve has been preserved, there is a very high chance it will recover completely. Postoperative cord assessment is advised at 2 days to determine whether there has been a permanent injury, but with transient bruising, the voice may take up to 6 months to recover fully. Meanwhile, treatment should be supportive, with nebulisers to lubricate the vocal cords and ongoing review with voice therapy as required. Only bilateral damage would necessitate an intervention to control the airway.

15. D 2% risk of permanent hypocalcaemia, 0.2% risk of permanent recurrent laryngeal nerve injury

The rate of recurrent nerve injury is quoted as 0.1% per lobectomy, performed in expert hands. For a total thyroidectomy, a reasonable assumption would be to double this risk. It is important to accurately identify the recurrent laryngeal nerve intraoperatively to minimise the risk of iatrogenic injury (**Figure 4.6**).

The risk of permanent hypocalcaemia requiring supplementation is around 2%. This is defined at 6 months postoperatively, after which time parathyroid function is unlikely to gain further in recovery. The risk of postoperative bleeding is approximately 2%, but not all cases will necessitate a return to theatre.

Relative bruising and ischaemia may explain the transient, minor symptoms experienced by patients, but does not equate to a nerve palsy caused by severing the nerve.

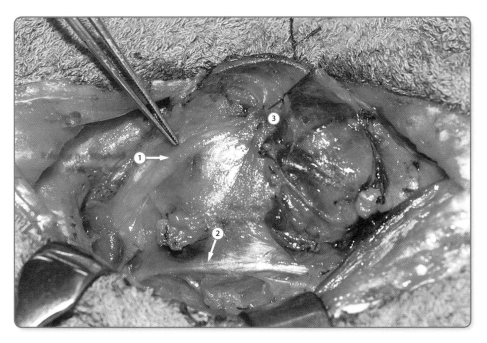

Figure 4.6 Intraoperative view of an exposed recurrent laryngeal nerve. ①Inferior parathyroid in upper horn thyrmus, ②recurrent laryngeal nerve, ③left lobe thyroid.

16. A Diagnostic lobectomy

This patient has an isolated swelling, which should be removed by diagnostic lobectomy. Despite the cystic nature of the lesion, given its size (and the patient's age), a resection is recommended. Ultrasound may allow temporisation, although only if reassuring features can be demonstrated (e.g. a well-defined isoechoic lesion). The risks of underlying malignancy as estimated by clinical characteristics, applicable to all such patients, are shown in **Figure 4.7**.

The sex of the patient, and nature of the swelling and the thyroid gland may be used to attribute a risk estimate to guide further investigations and management. Male

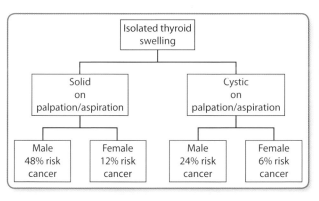

Figure 4.7 The risk of malignancy in palpable thyroid swellings, as defined by 30 years' prospective audit in a single specialist unit.

sex, and solid, isolated nodules are the most suspicious; women with dominant cystic swellings having the lowest risk. The risk of underlying malignancy in any generalised thyroid swelling is quoted at 3% within the same series.

17. C Nodes (1 cm) at level IV on the right

For patients presenting with a tumour of this size with no nodal disease, a total thyroidectomy and diagnostic central compartment dissection is deemed the appropriate treatment. Were lymph nodes involved in the central compartment, both sides would require clearance and hence a 'therapeutic' dissection. In option E these lesions may well be benign, measuring <1 cm, but should be explored anyway. Ultrasound alone has a poor positive predictive value for malignancy, but 70% accuracy overall. Therefore, with a pre-existing diagnosis, this plan will not alter. Multinodular disease would strengthen the case in favour of a total thyroidectomy over a lobectomy, were the tumour to be smaller. Nodes at level IV, if likely to be involved as indicated by size criteria, imply that the lateral compartment may be positive for disease. Biopsy should be obtained and a unilateral modified neck dissection carried out in addition to the planned procedure if disease is confirmed pre- or perioperatively.

18. D 85%

The majority of patients with sporadic hyperparathyroidism have a single adenoma (85%), with 13% having a four-gland hyperplasia, and the minority having more than one adenoma, or a carcinoma. The parathyroid hormone level does not correlate well with the size of the gland. Multiple adenomas are found more frequently in older patients. Cancers are characteristically adhesive, larger and sometimes obviously invasive. With lack of positive imaging in this patient, she should still have the other side of her neck explored, but there is a high chance that this is her only source of upset, and removal will lead to cure.

19. B Serum calcitonin

Calcitonin is the single most useful marker of medullary disease, with tumours derived from the parafollicular C-cells. It is classically used as a quantitative tumour marker both pre- and postoperatively. Although there is interaction, particularly on immunohistochemistry, with carcinoid tumours, chromogranin A alone is not used as a standard marker. Carcinoembryonic antigen may be elevated, and is sometimes used as a diagnostic screen test for medullary disease, whereas other elements of the medullary endocrine neoplasia-2A syndrome may lead to an elevated serum calcium level. Thyroglobulin is useful for the follow-up of patients who have already undergone resection or suppression for cancer. With patients who still have a normal thyroid in situ, there is no utility for this as a diagnostic test.

20. E Size of the lesion

This CT has identified an adrenal incidentaloma. These are an increasingly common finding with the volume of radiological images being performed in modern practice. Tumour size is the most significant factor alone in distinguishing benign and malignant lesions. Primary adrenocortical carcinoma occurs in 2% of tumours <4 cm, but in 25% of those which are >6 cm. Consequently, those >4 cm should be considered at highest risk, and therefore their removal is advocated. Lesion homo- or heterogeneity is unreliable, and although functional tests must be carried out on all such lesions prior to intervention, results of these, along with patient age and sex, cannot be taken in isolation to predict reliably malignant potential.

21. E There is a 5% chance that this lesion is a phaeochromocytoma

This is the correct, representative risk of phaeochromocytoma, which is an important diagnosis of exclusion in any incidentaloma. Thirty per cent of phaeochromocytoma cases are diagnosed from incidentalomas, not 50% as in option A. At <4 cm, the risk of malignancy is < 2%. Adrenal lesions notoriously present late, with significant enlargement required for any symptoms to arise from this retroperitoneal organ, normally in the form of pressure on adjacent organs, rather than pain. In the absence of positive functional tests, and insufficient size criteria to be concerned about malignancy, the scan should be repeated at a 6-month interval to determine the growth characteristics which may further determine the need for surgery.

22. E Ultrasound scan, FNAC of thyroid and nodal scan

This patient probably has a diagnosis of papillary thyroid PTC. Ultrasound-guided fine-needle aspiration cytology (FNAC) has the highest sensitivity for diagnosis at first attempt, and the patient will also require a scan to assess the nodes. If these are suspicious, further FNAC should be performed to guide the extent of surgery required. If papillary thyroid cancer is confirmed and the grade is THY5, he should also undergo a chest X-ray to rule out further metastases.

Answers: EMIs

23. A Adrenocortical carcinoma

The family history in this scenario is typical of Li–Fraumeni mutation, and in the available list of tumours, adrenocortical carcinoma is most likely to be associated with the syndrome. If a patient is diagnosed with adrenocortical cancer at a young age, some argue that this diagnosis alone is sufficient to warrant genetic testing for Li–Fraumeni syndrome. It is driven by inactivation of the tumour suppressor gene p53. These patients are also predisposed to brain tumours.

24. H Parathyroid adenoma

In multiple endocrine neoplasia-1 (MEN-1) syndrome, patients suffer from parathyroid, pancreatic and pituitary tumours (in this order of frequency). Thus, this man requires a calcium/parathyroid hormone profile, and if both are raised, further imaging must be organised so that appropriate parathyroid surgery can be planned. In MEN-1, even if only one gland is apparently abnormal, there is a strong argument for total parathyroidectomy given that the other glands are likely to undergo change, with typically 3 or 4 glands involved. There is a tendency to recurrence following subtotal parathyroidectomy. Primary hyperparathyroidism is present in at least 90% of MEN-1 patients aged >50 years, and is the most common initial clinical presentation.

25. D Medullary carcinoma of the thyroid

In this patient's case, his father has presented with medullary thyroid carcinoma (MTC) at a late stage with metastatic disease. This probably represents a new mutation within the multiple endocrine neoplasia-2A (MEN-2A) category. These patients have normal bodily habitus, unlike the 2B patients, but are at risk of medullary thyroid cancer, as well as parathyroid disease and phaeochromocytoma. Decisions on the timing of surgery in new cases of MEN-2 (without apparent MTC at presentation) are carried out in a risk-stratified fashion, based on known genotype-phenotype relationships of the different RET (the REarranged in Transfection proto-oncogene, a tyrosine kinase receptor gene) mutations. The highest risk patients should have a thyroidectomy within their first year of life.

26. F THY5 (malignant) on fine-needle aspiration cytology

This woman probably has a primary papillary thyroid cancer (PTC), which despite probable lymph node involvement, carries an excellent prognosis because of her age, sex and the size of the tumour. She needs to undergo total thyroidectomy with lymph node surgery determined by preoperative ultrasound imaging. The single most important diagnostic test is a fine-needle aspiration cytology (FNAC) of the primary lesion which, if reported as THY5, is consistent with definitive evidence of malignancy, and the operation will go ahead as outlined for THY1–5 breakdown, which is the standard reporting mechanism for FNAC.

For thyroid FNAC, there are five simplified scores, as described in the guidelines for the management of thyroid cancer (British Thyroid Association, 2014). Subsequent divisions are possible, e.g. THY1C if the aspirate is cystic, yielding >1 mL fluid; for exam purposes, this level of knowledge, and subsequent management recommendations is adequate.

27. D None of these options

This man's phaeochromocytoma may be subject to complex histopathology reporting, including chromogranin A (consistent with neuroendocrine tumours) and the full Weiss criteria (**Table 4.3**) which details nine different histological features. However, the only definitive marker of malignancy in phaeochromocytoma is the development of distant metastases, and because none of the listed criteria here are the most relevant, follow-up remains clinical.

Table 4.3 Histological assessment of neuroendocrine tumours: Weiss criteria

Weiss criteria

- High mitotic rate
- High nuclear grade
- Low percentage clear cells
- Necrosis
- Diffuse architecture of tumour
- Capsular invasion
- Sinusoidal invasion
- Venous invasion
- Atypical mitoses

Each feature present is worth a score of 1.
- Total <2 = adenoma
- Total >3 = malignancy

None are definitive alone for malignancy, but the score progressively indicates a higher risk tumour
Adapted from Weiss LM. Comparative histologic study of 43 metastasizing and nonmetastasizing adrenocortical tumours. Am J Pathol 1984; 8:163–169.

28. A C-cell hyperplasia

This case probably represents a sporadic medullary carcinoma and in the absence of a genetic mutation, the risk of recurrence and of the cancer being inherited by offspring is negligible. Ordinarily, the clinical marker of this is the absence of C-cell hyperplasia in the remaining resected thyroid gland.

29. B Chronic lymphocytic thyroiditis (Hashimoto's disease)

This patient probably has chronic lymphocytic thyroiditis, whereby the lymphocytic infiltration of the thyroid (**Figure 4.8**), with a secondary inflammatory response, leads to a moderate enlargement of the thyroid and a characteristically 'bosselated' feel. Chronically, low circulating thyroid hormone levels will also stimulate growth of the gland (**Figure 4.9**) and this condition is associated with positive thyroid autoantibodies.

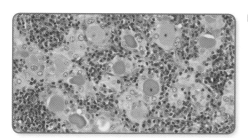

Figure 4.8 Histopathology of thyroiditis.

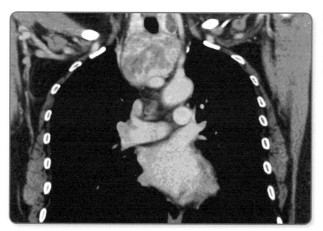

Figure 4.9 Typical appearances of a multinodular goitre, seen on coronal sections at CT. This need not be associated with any specific thyroiditis.

30. C de Quervain's thyroiditis

This is de Quervain's thyroiditis (Hashimoto's disease) which characteristically occurs following an upper respiratory tract infection, and commonly leads to pain on swallowing. The symptoms may last several weeks before spontaneous resolution. Treatment is supportive with non-steroidal anti-inflammatory drugs, and, if associated with transient hyperthyroidism, beta-blockers may be used. Severe cases may require treatment with steroids.

31. H Riedel's thyroiditis

This case represents Riedel's thyroiditis. This condition is more common among the women, and is associated with a 'woody hard' swelling in the thyroid as an isolated abnormality. Surgical relief of compressive symptoms is sometimes required if treatment with high dose steroids is not effective (and is necessary if the differential diagnosis of anaplastic carcinoma cannot be ruled out). Thyroxine replacement is also required. Riedel's thyroiditis accounts for only 0.5% of all goitres.

32. C Lobectomy alone then thyroid-stimulating hormone (TSH) suppression

This scenario describes a low-risk papillary microcarcinoma, with no adverse risk factors present. The patient is young and female with a small, likely incidental cancer, and no evidence of metastatic or extrathyroidal disease. In such patients, lobectomy alone and subsequent TSH suppression represents adequate therapy. The disease is effectively an incidental entity. In general terms, the well-described risk stratification systems by the Mayo Clinic (2002) may be used to guide the extent of treatment, although with a lack of consistent level 1 and 2 evidence, the lack of guideline consensus persists.

33. D Radioiodine treatment following appropriate surgery to the neck

This presentation is of metastatic follicular cancer. This differentiated tumour type tends to present in a slightly older age group than papillary disease. There is a tendency for haematogenous rather than nodal spread, and presentations with metastases are not uncommon (**Figure 4.10**). Having dealt with symptomatic metastases, optimal treatment involves total thyroidectomy (irrespective of clinical findings in the neck) in order that radioiodine may be administered and taken up by metastatic disease. Without thyroidectomy the compound would simply concentrate in the neck. Typically, the tumour retains enough differentiation to allow a reasonable expectation of symptomatic benefit from this, with a corresponding fall in thyroglobulin expected.

Haematogenous spread is near specific to this form of differentiated thyroid cancer.

34. A Debulking surgery then external beam radiation therapy

This patient has advanced anaplastic thyroid cancer. This carries a rapidly fatal prognosis, and is typically unresponsive to chemotherapy. The best treatment for local control is external beam therapy, but if the patient presents with locally compressive symptoms and airway compromise (and in this case with a high likelihood of recurrent laryngeal nerve involvement), basic decompressive surgery (e.g. isthmusectomy) is a reasonable first step before administering the necessary radiation. More extensive surgery is not warranted, as therapy will not be curative, and the risk of damaging a functional nerve is too great.

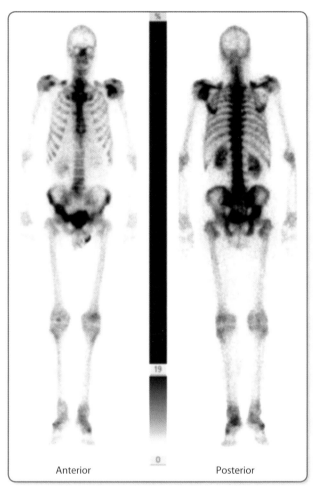

Figure 4.10 Follicular carcinoma presenting with bony metastases.

Anterior   Posterior

35. F Repeat CT scanning at annual interval(s)

This scenario describes a classical 'incidentaloma'. A lesion which, but for CT, we would not know existed, and which is extremely unlikely to cause any harm. Myolipomas are benign growths related to the adrenal gland, and even when size criteria would otherwise suggest excision is necessary (≥4 cm), with appropriate radiological expertise in reporting, with or without supplementary MRI, it is possible to leave these lesions in situ. CT imaging as seen in **Figure 4.11** can identify neoplastic lesions which will require urgent treatment. In this patient's case, with a lesion this size a repeat CT in 1 year's time would be the best management plan.

This lesion is in contrast to an 'incidentaloma'. Here the heterogeneous nature and enormous size makes a diagnosis of carcinoma a certainty.

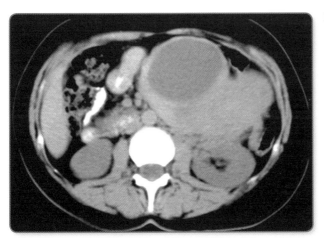

Figure 4.11 Adrenal mass on CT.

36. A CT-guided biopsy

Given this woman's history, the most important diagnosis of exclusion is metastatic cancer. Although it is important to perform urinary tests to exclude a phaeochromocytoma before making any intervention, the single most important test in this woman's case is a tissue diagnosis to exclude or diagnose metastatic breast carcinoma. Caution must be applied, however, to determine if there is any possible hormonal component, and so urinary metanephrine and catecholamine collections would also be carried out. Clinically silent phaeochromocytoma are not uncommon and necessitate these investigations, so that any intervention may be carried out safely.

37. B Dexamethasone suppression test

This man probably has bilateral cortical adenomas as a cause for hypertension driven by Cushing's disease. Around 15% patients with incidentalomas have bilateral lesions, and these are most commonly cortical adenomas, metastatic disease, or congenital adrenal hyperplasia. The scenario makes no mention of systemic illness, other hormonal problems or longer standing concerns. Thus, in the context of hypertension, this is the most likely explanation. With a borderline cortisol rise, the definitive investigation is a dexamethasone suppression test.

38. I Tertiary hyperparathyroidism

This rare condition occurs in patients who have been in chronic renal failure, but who have recovered their renal function post-transplant. Autonomous parathyroid function, because of the constant hypocalcaemia in the context of renal hyperphosphataemia, has 'reset' the parathyroid glands so that they continue to produce parathyroid hormone without the normal feedback inhibition, which results in hypercalcaemia. There is a 60% chance of resolution spontaneously, but, if it persists beyond 12 months it is normally severe, and requires total parathyroidectomy.

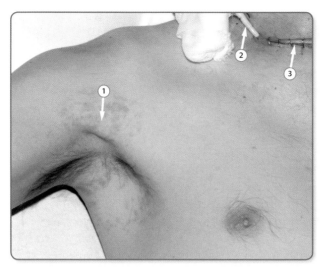

Figure 4.12 Calciphylaxis. Soft tissue deposition of calcium which can constitute a surgical emergency. ① Skin rash of calciphylaxis, ② dialysis catheter, ③ incision for total parathyroidectomy.

In this patient's case, calciphylaxis has resulted (**Figure 4.12**). This patient is seen postoperatively where he remains dialysis dependent, having undergone an unsuccessful renal transplantation.

Here, soft tissue and vascular calcification can lead to tissue necrosis; it is found most commonly in the extremities and is associated with a significant mortality rate. It is treated by phosphate binders and urgent parathyroidectomy. Patients with a high calcium and phosphorous product are most at risk (i.e. patients with recovered renal function but persistent hypercalcaemia).

39. G Primary hyperparathyroidism

This is a typical case of primary hyperparathyroidism (PHP), picked up only as a consequence of osteoporosis screening (in the context of a fracture in the elderly female population). The true incidence of PHP is unknown. Anecdotally, regions where routine calcium level testing is performed on the 'urea and electrolyte' admission blood profile have a higher incidence. It is a fair assumption that the condition is under-diagnosed, and only a minority present with the typical hypercalcaemic picture of renal calculi, abdominal pain, and psychiatric disturbance. Following the diagnosis (by way of serum biochemistry) appropriate imaging investigations will be performed to attempt to localise the source (87–90% due to single gland adenoma, 3% multiple adenomas, 9% four-gland hyperplasia and 1% carcinoma).

40. C Multiple endocrine neoplasia-1 (MEN-1) syndrome

This patient has two problems from the spectrum of possible conditions within MEN-1 syndrome (a pancreatic glucagonoma and hyperparathyroidism, normally consisting of four-gland hyperplasia). Both MEN-1 and MEN-2A syndromes are associated with hyperparathyroidism, but it is more aggressive in the former. The choice must be made between total parathyroidectomy with lifelong calcium supplementation or a subtotal parathyroidectomy (leaving a tiny remnant in the neck or utilising autotransplantation). Both of the latter options risk the need for reoperative surgery and increased perioperative morbidity.

41. I Phaeochromocytoma

This patient probably has MEN-2A, the common associations being medullary thyroid carcinoma (in 90%), phaeochromocytoma (in 50%) and primary hyperparathyroidism (in 30%). Adrenal lesions are less commonly seen in MEN-1, and in the absence of other endocrine symptoms, MEN-2A should be the working diagnosis.

He will require clinical assessment of his thyroid, with a serum calcitonin, as well as a full work up for this probable phaeochromocytoma. Given his age, he represents a sporadic, new mutation (as a member of the recognised kindred would have had resulted in full screening investigations carried out in childhood). In this context, phaeochromocytoma can be unilateral or bilateral, and in aggressive phenotypes, can even present in the first decade of life. It is important to exclude phaeochromocytoma in any established MEN-associated disease, prior to surgery for any linked, or even separate, condition. Plasma metanephrines alone may generate false negatives, and urinary collections remain important.

42. C Gastrinoma

This woman has primary hyperparathyroidism and probably a gastrinoma underlying her gastrointestinal presentation. Her symptoms can all be explained by multiple endocrine neoplasia-1 (MEN-1) syndrome. Her father also seemed to have suffered from parathyroid and probable pancreatic neuroendocrine disease. In addition, hypercalcaemia will contribute to peptic ulcer disease. Gastrinomas within MEN-1 are often multifocal and small, and can be situated in the duodenum. Pathology driven by these will respond to proton pump inhibitor treatment, but the acid hypersecretion will persist. Surgery for gastrinoma in MEN-1 is frequently not curative, and may be extensive (e.g. Whipple's procedure). Patients with markers of aggressive disease at presentation have a poorer outcome, associated with decreased survival, and they warrant consideration of more aggressive treatment.

Diagnosis of MEN-1:

- <35 years of age
- Onset of gastrinoma <27 years of age
- Markedly elevated gastrin at presentation
- Tumour size >3 cm

43. E Insulinoma

This patient has symptoms suggestive of an insulinoma within multiple endocrine neoplasia-1 (MEN-1) syndrome. Primary hyperparathyroidism alone does not always trigger a hunt for other associated diagnoses, although in such a young patient, we assume some thought was given to this at initial presentation. There is now a suggested schema for screening such patients in order to make timely diagnoses and interventions (summarised in **Table 4.4**).

This schema represents a programme for biochemical and radiological follow-up of MEN-1 patients – Ball et al. (2009) provides more details. For islet cell tumours, anterior pituitary, and foregut carcinoids, MRI should be performed as appropriate at 3–5 yearly intervals.

Table 4.4 MEN-1 associations and routine biochemical investigations		
Tumour type	**Investigations**	**Frequency of test**
Parathyroid adenoma	Ca^{2+} Parathyroid hormone	Annual
Enteropancreatic islet cell	Gastrin Glucose Insulin Vasoactive intestinal peptide Pancreatic polypeptide Glucagon Somatostatin	Annual
Anterior pituitary	Prolactin Insulin like growth factor-1	Annual
Foregut carcinoid	Chromogranin A	Annual

44. J Thyroglossal cyst

This is a classical description of a thyroglossal cyst, which is quite a separate entity from a thyroid gland swelling per se. It results from persistence of part of the thyroglossal duct, and although embryologically midline, may be felt slightly to one or other side, just below the hyoid. Movement upwards on swallowing is diagnostic, with superior movement on tongue protrusion the result of its attachment to the foramen caecum (**Figure 4.13**). These frequently present with infection – hence, the erythema noted in the scenario. For this reason alone, thyroglossal cysts are best excised, by way of a Sistrunk procedure, which formally excises part of the hyoid bone. Inadequate removal or persistent infections can result in thyroglossal fistulae at a lower level in the neck than the original cyst. They classically present in childhood or early adulthood.

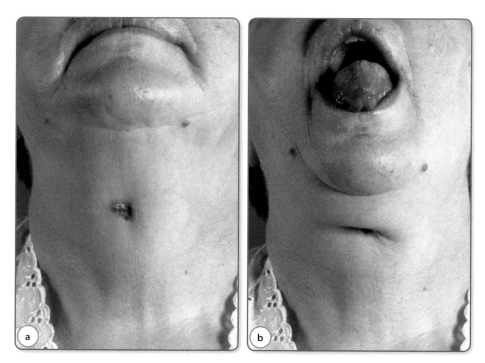

Figure 4.13 Typical appearances of a midline cyst, which rises on protrusion of the tongue. This cyst has fistulated with chronic infection.

45. H Pharyngeal pouch

In this scenario featuring a middle-aged woman, it may be tempting to attribute the diagnosis of 'globus hystericus' (where there is no substantive pathology and anxiety leads to dysphagia). However, the history of food regurgitation is characteristic of a pharyngeal pouch, and although there is no visible or palpable abnormality in the neck, it is not unusual for such patients to present to the thyroid clinic. A contrast swallow should be arranged to further investigate symptoms in the first instance (**Figure 4.14**).

46. E Metastatic papillary carcinoma

Despite this patient's smoking history, given her age, sex, and the obvious extent of disease, the likely diagnosis is papillary thyroid cancer with metastatic spread to lymph nodes. The appearances are consistent with a primary tumour situated within the thyroid gland. Despite the nodal disease, at this patient's young age curative surgery is still very likely, with a 20-year survival rate of 98%; at age < 45 years, nodal disease is still classified as Stage I overall. This is entirely different to a patient presenting with locally extensive squamous disease, the surgical management of which requires a completely different, radical approach.

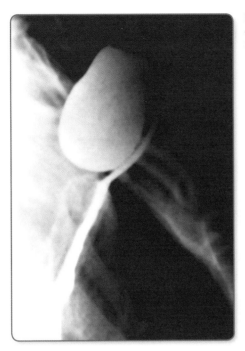

Figure 4.14 Typical fluoroscopic appearances of a pharyngeal pouch, leading to characteristic regurgitation and halitosis.

47. A 5-Hydroxyindoleacetic acid level.

Carcinoid syndrome is a paraneoplastic syndrome secondary to carcinoid tumours. It classically produces symptoms of flushing and diarrhoea secondary to endogenous secretion of serotonin and kallikrein. If the primary tumour is from the GI tract usually carcinoid syndrome does not occur until the disease is so advanced that the liver cannot metabolise serotonin. Abdominal pain is usually caused by liver metastases. 24-hour urine collection to measure 5-hydroxyindoleacetic acid (the end product of serotonin metabolism) levels should be checked.

48. D Gastrin

Zollinger–Ellison syndrome is caused by a non-β islet cell, gastrin-secreting tumour of the pancreas that stimulates gastric acid secretion leading to gastrointestinal mucosal ulceration. Zollinger–Ellison syndrome is sporadic in 75% of patients, whereas in the other 25% it is associated with MEN 1, an autosomal dominant condition characterised by hyperparathyroidism, pancreatic endocrine tumours, and pituitary tumours. Serum gastrin levels should be taken in the fasting state. Raised serum calcium levels would raise the suspicion of MEN 1.

49. I Vanillylmandelic acid level

Phaeochromocytoma is a neuroendocrine tumour of the medulla of the adrenal gland, originating in the chromaffin cells. It secretes chatecholamines (noradrenaline and adrenaline). Vanillylmandelic acid and is an end-stage metabolite of adrenaline and noradrenaline and is measured in a 24-hour urine collection. Phaeochromocytoma is part of the MEN 2A and B syndromes.

50. A Cinacalcet treatment

This patient is unfit for surgery. With secondary hyperparathyroidism and four-gland hyperplasia, a total parathyroidectomy via formal exploration would normally be a reasonable step, but in this case it may be better avoided. The NICE guideline TA117 (NICE; 2007) is specific to such patients. Cinacalcet is a calcimimetic that is a treatment option for patients who cannot undergo surgery. It acts by increasing the sensitivity of calcium receptors to extracellular calcium, thus preventing release of parathyroid hormone. It is recommended for treatment of refractory secondary hyperparathyroidism in patients with end-stage renal disease. This is the case even for patients with calciphylaxis, if they have uncontrolled levels of parathyroid hormone with normal or high adjusted calcium, and when surgery is contraindicated. A response to treatment is required as continuing treatment beyond 4 months is only advised if the parathyroid hormone level reduces by ≥30%.

51. I Targeted excision of one gland

This patient's investigations have been consistent with a solitary parathyroid adenoma causing primary hyperparathyroidism. With concordant imaging, she is a particularly good candidate for a targeted approach. Alone, a positive ultrasound has 80% sensitivity, a sestamibi has 92% sensitivity, and in combination sensitivity approaches 98%. The question of operative approach includes targeted open (consisting of a 3 cm lateral incision) and endoscopic procedures, and the decision is in part best addressed through local expertise. The majority of surgeons would prefer to take a conventional approach, and are less likely to have been specifically trained in endoscopic techniques (which routinely use a 2 cm midline incision). There may be further argument for endoscopic approach if the adenoma site was less certain, allowing full exploration on the side in question, or even contralaterally.

52. F No treatment, review in 1 year

In this scenario, the patient probably has primary hyperparathyroidism, but in the absence of symptoms, and a calcium level remaining at <2.8 mmol/L, there is no urgency for treatment. This is reinforced by his recent myocardial infarction, making general anaesthetic within the 3 months postevent window a further contraindication. With discordant imaging, he would require formal exploration, whereas only a minority of surgeons would attempt an open, targeted approach to a solitary lesion under local anaesthetic anyway. Although there is no strict biochemical evidence for a cut-off point at which parathyroidectomy becomes mandatory, there is now evidence to show improved outcomes in terms of long term musculoskeletal and cardiovascular morbidity when it is treated. Once this man has stabilised, a formal surgical approach may be advised.

Chapter 5

Hepatobiliary surgery

Questions: SBAs

For each question, select the single best answer from the five options listed.

1. A 28-year-old woman, who is 18 weeks pregnant, presents to her GP with intermittent right upper quadrant pain and dyspepsia. Her partner reports that she looked 'yellow' 1 week ago, but she does not currently appear jaundiced. She is generally well, apyrexial, and she is able to maintain normal dietary intake. A scan performed at the GP surgery confirms gallstones, without evidence of cholecystitis, and the common bile duct measures 6 mm, within normal limits. Bilirubin, amylase and liver function tests are all normal.

    What is the most appropriate management?

    A   Dietary advice and nothing more for now
    B   Laparoscopic cholecystectomy on the next available list
    C   List and defer for laparoscopic cholecystectomy once the baby is delivered
    D   Magnetic resonance cholangiopancreatography (MRCP)
    E   Open cholecystectomy

2. A 62-year-old man presents as a general surgical emergency with jaundice, associated with anorexia, low-grade fever, early satiety and weight loss. He had gallstones 20 years ago, which were managed by way of sphincterotomy and he has had no interim problems, being otherwise fit and well.

    What is the most appropriate investigation?

    A   Abdominal ultrasound
    B   CT of the abdomen
    C   Endoscopic ultrasound examination
    D   Endoscopic retrograde cholangiopancreatography
    E   Magnetic resonance cholangiopancreatography

3. A 40-year-old woman presents for a second time with cholecystitis, without biochemical evidence of pancreatitis; ultrasounds have previously demonstrated calculi within the gallbladder, and a normal, 7 mm duct. On this admission, her bilirubin is mildly elevated, at 40 μmol/L, with liver transaminases also slightly deranged. The bilirubin falls within normal limits by 24 hours, but her abdomen continues to be tender, with elevated inflammatory markers on intravenous antibiotics.

    What is the most appropriate intervention?

    A Endoscopic retrograde cholangiogram with sphincterotomy and balloon trawl
    B Laparoscopic cholecystectomy only
    C Laparoscopic cholecystectomy with on-table cholangiogram
    D Magnetic resonance cholangiogram
    E Re-admit at 6 weeks for laparoscopic cholecystectomy

4. A 46-year-old man with a 13 kg weight loss undergoes a CT of his abdomen which diagnoses cancer in the head of the pancreas.

    Which of the following statements best describes the management of pancreatic cancer?

    A All patients should undergo endoscopic ultrasound assessment of a suspected lesion
    B Pylorus-preserving pancreaticoduodenectomy may be the preferred treatment option for patients with advanced disease
    C Surgical options do not exist for locally advanced disease
    D Triple phase CT of the abdomen reliably stages the lymph nodes
    E Tumours are chemoradiation resistant with few palliative options

5. A 65-year-old man undergoing abdominal ultrasound scan is diagnosed with hepatocellular carcinoma (HCC).

    Which of the following statements best describes primary HCC?

    A α-Fetoprotein and CT should be used as screening tools at regular intervals
    B HCC screening is of value in the general population
    C Hepatitis B virus is more carcinogenic than hepatitis C virus
    D Men are relatively more at risk of HCC than women
    E Most patients with HCC are part of screening programs and have early, resectable disease.

6. A 44-year-old woman, who underwent a right hemicolectomy for caecal carcinoma, is identified on follow-up scan to have developed metastatic liver lesions.

    Which of the following statements best describes the selection of patients for liver resection in the context of colorectal cancer metastases?

    A Metastases should not be resected if surgery is only feasible following downstaging with chemotherapy
    B Patients should only be considered if all lesions can be managed synchronously
    C Patients with recurrent metastases (following limited resection) cannot be considered for further surgery
    D Previous chemotherapy administration may limit the extent of surgery offered
    E Radiofrequency ablation may facilitate resection of liver lesions, without significant associated risk

7. A 60-year-old man presents as a general surgical emergency with severe pancreatitis.

    Which of the following statements best describes the severity of acute severe pancreatitis?

    A Body mass index correlates poorly with severity
    B Severe pancreatitis is defined as organ(s) failure and/or local pancreatic complications
    C Severe pancreatitis is initially predicted from the Glasgow–Imrie score ≥ 3
    D Severity is not judged on the same criteria as other organ scoring systems
    E Severity may only be scored at 48 hours

8. A 54-year-old woman presents as a general surgical emergency with mild acute pancreatitis.

    Which of the following statements does not describe the aetiology of acute pancreatitis in the Western world?

    A Alcohol accounts for approximately 25% of cases, with approximately 10% of alcoholics developing acute pancreatitis
    B Gallstones account for approximately 35% of cases, with approximately 15% of patients developing acute pancreatitis
    C 'Idiopathic' pancreatitis should only account for approximately 20% of all cases
    D Mumps virus, cytomegalovirus and HIV are all associated with pancreatitis
    E Small gallstones are more likely to cause an obstructive problem, leading to acute pancreatitis

9. A 66-year-old man presents with acute severe pancreatitis.

   Which of the following statements best describes the complications of acute pancreatitis?

   A   Empirical antibiotic therapy is recommended for pancreatic necrosis associated with ongoing pyrexia
   B   Immediate fine-needle aspiration of pancreatic necrosis >30% volume should be obtained
   C   Pancreatic pseudocysts requiring surgical drainage require an open approach
   D   Staged laparotomies with open abdominal wound management systems successfully manage pancreatic necrosis
   E   Sterile necrosis should be drained (surgically/radiologically); without drainage, the sequelae will be worse

10. A 49-year-old woman is an alcoholic who has developed chronic pancreatitis with marked pain.

    Which of the following statements best describes the management of pain in chronic pancreatitis?

    A   Endoscopic decompressive measures are rarely of benefit
    B   Low fat diets are helpful to relieve dietary pain
    C   Ongoing alcohol consumption should be primarily addressed, even in established pancreatitis
    D   Pancreatic enzyme supplementation is helpful in reducing dietary pain
    E   Total pancreatectomy is the surgical procedure of choice for pain refractory to other interventions

11. A 48-year-old woman presents to surgical outpatients with intermittent dyspepsia and right upper quadrant pain. 7 years ago she had a potentially curative mastectomy and right axillary clearance for a high-grade, T3N1 carcinoma of the breast. She underwent adjuvant chemotherapy and has remained well until now. The history is in keeping with biliary colic, and an abdominal ultrasound reveals three hypoechoic lesions within segments V and VI of the liver; she also has gallstones. A CT subsequently confirms appearances consistent with isolated metastases in the right lobe, without any other intra-abdominal pathology.

    What is the most appropriate management plan?

    A   Obtain a tissue diagnosis with core biopsy
    B   Obtain a tissue diagnosis with fine-needle aspiration cytology
    C   Refer to the hepatobiliary and pancreatic surgeons for a limited right hepatectomy
    D   Refer to medical oncology for consideration of chemotherapy
    E   Watchful waiting

12. A 51-year-old man has a neuroendocrine tumour diagnosed by his GP.

Which of the following statements best describes gut neuroendocrine tumours?

A   Serum chromogranin and urinary 5-hydroxyindoleacetic acid levels are useful in the diagnosis

B   The majority of tumours become symptomatic quickly

C   They are frequently part of a familial syndrome of multiple endocrine neoplasia

D   They constitute a straightforward diagnosis

E   They do not present with hormonal symptoms until very advanced

13. A 27-year-old woman undergoes an emergency splenectomy following a fall whilst horse riding.

Which of the following statements best describes her perioperative care?

A   All patients require full cross-match preparation with platelets available

B   The incidence of postoperative sepsis is negligible in the absence of malignant disease

C   Vaccinations must be administered prior to the patient leaving hospital

D   Vaccinations should be administered within the first 2 weeks postsurgery

E   Vaccinations should include polyvalent pneumococcus, *Haemophilus influenzae B* and meningococcus

14. A 54-year-old man with thrombocytopaenia requires an elective splenectomy. He is interested in the various surgical options. Which of the following statements best describes the operative procedure of splenectomy?

A   At open splenectomy, all the hilar vessels require individual control

B   Laparoscopic splenectomy is a safe option in immune thrombocytopaenic purpura

C   Laparoscopic splenectomy has become the standard approach

D   Laparoscopic splenectomy has the same rate of postoperative complications as open operation

E   Open splenectomy is always the operation of choice in moderate splenomegaly

15. A 72-year-old man presents as an emergency with haematemesis. He is diagnosed with oesophageal varices secondary to portal hypertension.

Which of the following statements best describes the treatment of portal hypertension?

A   Beta-blockade prevents re-bleeding in a proportion, but does not reduce overall mortality

B   It can never be cured by splenectomy

C   Overall mortality is reduced with ongoing beta-blockade

D   Pharmacological treatment reduces bleeding risk from 25% to 15% in patients with varices

E   Prevention of varices requires propranolol for patients with cirrhosis and abnormal portal venous flow

16. A 27-year-old woman sustains an injury to her common bile duct during laparoscopic cholecystectomy.

Which of the following statements best describes the classification of injuries to the common bile duct?

A   A cystic duct stump leak is included in formal classification systems
B   Injuries described by Strasberg A, B and C criteria rarely require formal intervention
C   Injury resulting in no residual liver drainage is outwith formal classification
D   The Bismuth classification can be used during surgery to describe the injury
E   The Strasberg classification describes four types of injury, with subclassification within some categories

17. A 42-year-old woman sustains an iatrogenic bile duct injury during laparoscopic cholecystectomy.

Which of the following statements best describes the management of injury to the biliary tree?

A   A ductal T-tube and a subhepatic drain offer a temporising measure before definitive management
B   Bile in an abdominal drain 48 hours postcholecystectomy is within normal acceptable limits
C   Endoscopic retrograde cholangiogram is always diagnostic of the degree of injury
D   Low straight-forward common bile duct injuries recognised at laparoscopic cholecystectomy should be repaired with primary suture
E   Significant biliary injuries managed in hepatobiliary units normally fully recover with minimal morbidity

18. A 64-year-old woman undergoes a CT of her abdomen which is highly suggestive of gallbladder malignancy.

Which of the following statements best describes primary neoplasia of the gallbladder?

A   A 'porcelain gallbladder' (with a calcified wall) mandates an urgent cholecystectomy
B   Adenomatous polyps of the gallbladder measuring <3 cm may be followed with serial ultrasounds
C   Cholecystoenteric fistula is a risk factor for malignancy
D   If gallbladder cancer is suspected (precholecystectomy) a tissue diagnosis must be obtained
E   Multiple polyps are more reassuring than a solitary, suspicious polyp

19. A 70-year-old woman with obstructive jaundice is diagnosed with cholangiocarcinoma.

Which of the following statements best describes cholangiocarcinoma?

A 5-year survival rates of 25–40% exist for those undergoing complete, curative resections

B Effective treatment options include chemoradiation for frail patients, or those with non-resectable disease

C Liver transplantation can be considered as a therapeutic option in an appropriate specialist centre

D No surgical options exist for locally advanced disease unlikely to achieve clear resection margins

E The overall prognosis of this tumour has seen marked improvement in recent times

Questions: EMIs

Theme: Treatment modalities

A　Best supportive care
B　Endoscopic retrograde cholangiopancreatography alone
C　Endoscopic retrograde cholangiopancreatography and sphincterotomy
D　Fine-needle aspiration of the pancreas then intravenous antibiotics

E　IV antibiotics
F　Laparoscopic cholecystectomy alone
G　Laparoscopic cholecystectomy and on-table cholangiogram
H　Open cholecystectomy
I　Total parenteral nutrition

Instructions: For each of the following scenarios, choose the single most likely treatment from the list above. Each option may be used once, more than once or not at all.

20.　A 41-year-old woman, with a body mass index of 37, presents with acute onset upper abdominal pain, associated with serum amylase 780 U/L, AAT 630 U/L and GGT 400 U/L. Her bilirubin is transiently elevated, and liver functions normalise by day 3 post-presentation. Magnetic resonance cholangiopancreatography (MRCP) demonstrates ductal dilatation (14 mm).

21.　An 82-year-old man is transferred to the hepatobiliary unit, having presented 10 days earlier with acute severe idiopathic pancreatitis. His liver function has normalised and he is not jaundiced, but he has ongoing fever, pain, and abdominal distension. A CT performed 2 days earlier demonstrates 35% pancreatic necrosis with a phlegmon.

22.　A 28-year-old woman, with documented gallstones, presents with acute pancreatitis, amylase 900 U/L, and contemporary MRCP confirms normal ductal anatomy. Her liver function has normalised by day 2.

Theme: Jaundice

A　Biliary stricture
B　Cholangiocarcinoma
C　Cholecystitis
D　Choledocholithiasis
E　Decompensated alcoholic liver disease

F　Fulminant liver failure
G　Head of pancreas tumour
H　Pancreatitis due to gallstones
I　Primary sclerosing cholangitis

Instructions: For each of the following scenarios, choose the single most likely diagnosis from the list above. Each option may be used once, more than once or not at all.

23.　A 30-year-old man, who has suffered ulcerative for over 15 years (resulting in a subtotal colectomy) presents acutely with painless jaundice and abdominal distension. His blood tests show bilirubin 150 μmol/L, AAT 400 U/L, GGT 900 U/L. The distension is due to ascites, but, his scan confirms normal gross hepatic parenchyma, but with reversed portal venous flow.

24.　A 59-year-old man presents with painless jaundice. He has no documented history of gallstones, and is otherwise well. On examination, a mass is palpable in the right upper quadrant. His blood profile shows an obstructive picture.

25. A 40-year-old woman presents with right upper quadrant pain, fevers, nausea and vomiting. Physical examination reveals mild jaundice, and a tender right upper quadrant. Her blood tests confirm a bilirubin rise of 60 µmol/L, AAT 120 U/L, GGT 110 U/L. On ultrasound, her common bile duct measures 8 mm.

Theme: Choledochal cysts (Todani classification)

A Type Ia
B Type Ib
C Type Ic
D Type II
E Type III
F Type IVa
G Type IVb
H Type V
I Type VI

Instructions: For each of the following scenarios choose the single most likely Todani classification from the list above. Each option may be used once, more than once or not at all.

26. Multiple dilatations/cysts involving only the extrahepatic bile duct.

27. Dilatation of the entire extrahepatic bile duct.

28. Multiple dilatations/cysts of the intrahepatic ducts only.

Theme: Liver neoplasia

A Chemotherapy
B Extended right hemihepatectomy
C External beam radiation
D Limited right hemihepatectomy
E Liver transplantation assessment
F Palliation – best supportive care
G Portal venous embolisation of tumour
H Radiofrequency ablation
I Wedge resection/segmentectomy

Instructions: For each of the following scenarios, choose the single most likely treatment from the list above. Each option may be used once, more than once or not at all.

29. A 65-year-old man with alcoholic liver disease, currently off alcohol for 2 years and on the screening programme, is diagnosed with bifocal hepatocellular carcinoma affecting segments IV/V and VII. Both nodules measure <3 cm. The entire liver is cirrhotic, but he has a normal bilirubin and prothrombin time with a Child–Pugh grade A.

30. A 60-year-old woman, with a background of hepatitis C, presents acutely with her first decompensation of chronic liver disease. An abdominal ultrasound confirms portal hypertension, and reports four foci of neoplastic disease affecting segments 7 and 8. She scores Child–Pugh grade B.

31. A 50-year-old woman is attending routine follow-up 3 years following a left hemihepatectomy for metastatic colorectal cancer. She had a previous Dukes stage C primary tumour resected at age 42 years. She is otherwise fit and well. A triple phase CT documents an isolated metastasis in segment VI which is confirmed by position emission tomography. Her synthetic liver function remains normal.

Theme: Benign liver lesions

A	Haemangioma	F	Liver abscess
B	Liver cell adenoma	G	Polycystic liver disease
C	Mesenchymal hamartoma	H	Focal nodular hyperplasia
D	Cyst adenoma	I	Nodular regenerative hyperplasia
E	Hydatid cyst		

Instructions: For each of the following scenarios, choose the single most likely diagnosis from the list above. Each option may be used once, more than once, or not at all

32. A 55-year-old woman presents with right upper quadrant pain. Ultrasound shows a 20-cm lesion which is anechoic.

33. An 18-month-old boy presents with abdominal distension and respiratory distress. Abdominal X-ray shows a noncalcified mass in the right upper quadrant. Abdominal ultrasound shows a multiseptated cystic lesion in the liver.

34. A 37-year-old woman presents with right upper quadrant pain. She has been taking the oral contraceptive pill for 17 years. Ultrasound imaging shows a well demarcated heterogenous hypervascular mass.

Theme: Neuroendocrine tumours

A	Appendiceal neuroendocrine tumour	F	Multiple endocrine neoplasia-1 (MEN-1) syndrome
B	Carcinoid syndrome		
C	Gastropancreatic carcinoid tumour	G	MEN-2 syndrome
D	Glucagonoma	H	VIPoma
E	Insulinoma	I	Zollinger–Ellison syndrome

Instructions: For each of the following scenarios, choose the single most likely diagnosis from the list above. Each option may be used once, more than once or not at all.

35. A 42-year-old woman, who has previously undergone a total parathyroidectomy for primary hyperparathyroidism, presents with weight loss and diarrhoea.

36. A 65-year-old man underwent appendicectomy necessitating completion right hemicolectomy 7 years earlier. He did not require any chemotherapy. He now presents with intermittent abdominal pain, diarrhoea and flushing.

37. A 56-year-old woman is undergoing investigations for unexplained abdominal pains. An upper gastrointestinal endoscopy demonstrated a prepyloric ulcer, and her symptoms have persisted despite taking proton pump inhibitors. A CT now reveals a small, homogenous mass in the tail of the pancreas.

Theme: Interventions for pancreatic cancer

A   Best supportive care
B   Endoscopic stenting of common bile duct (CBD) only
C   Endoscopic stenting of CBD and pancreatic duct
D   Laparoscopic enucleation of pancreatic tumour
E   Open bypass procedure: gastrojejunostomy
F   Open bypass procedure: hepaticojejunostomy
G   Pylorus-preserving pancreaticoduodenectomy
H   Referral for chemoradiation treatment
I   Whipple's procedure

Instructions: For each of the following scenarios, choose the single most likely treatment from the list above. Each option may be used once, more than once or not at all.

38. A 54-year-old man presents with painless jaundice (bilirubin >200 μmol/L) and is found on CT to have 'double duct dilatation' and features suggesting a pancreatic head mass. There is no obvious lymphadenopathy but further staging information is awaited, and will take over 2 weeks to arrange.

39. A 73-year-old woman with few comorbidities presents with epigastric pain, early satiety and vomiting; she has lost 6 kg in weight. Investigations are consistent with a locally advanced tumour in the pancreatic head/body. Her biliary drainage is uncompromised.

40. An 80-year-old man is diagnosed with locally advanced pancreatic cancer with portal vein involvement, but no compromise to biliary or gastric drainage. He wishes for 'something to be done'.

Theme: Portal hypertension

A   Acute alcoholic hepatitis
B   Budd–Chiari syndrome
C   Constrictive pericarditis
D   Haemochromatosis
E   Myelofibrosis
F   Portal vein thrombosis
G   Post viral cirrhotic disease
H   Primary biliary cirrhosis
I   Primary sclerosing cholangitis
J   Sarcoidosis

Instructions: For each of the following scenarios, choose the single most likely diagnosis from the list above. Each option may be used once, more than once or not at all.

41. A 26-year-old woman presents to acute medical receiving with jaundice and abdominal pain. On examination, she has ascites and is coagulopathic. CT demonstrates unusual liver perfusion. She has been on the oral contraceptive pill for 7 years.

42. A 63-year-old woman has undergone 2 weeks of aggressive, conservative (non-resectional) management for locally contained, perforated diverticulitis. Her condition has improved substantially. However, her liver function has become dramatically deranged, with a rise in bilirubin and evidence of coagulopathy. She complains of new, upper abdominal discomfort.

43. A 56-year-old man, with type 1 diabetes, presents to his GP with increasing abdominal distension, discomfort, easy bruising and general malaise. He is examined, and found to have splenomegaly and ascites, without obvious hepatomegaly.

Theme: Hepatobiliary sepsis

A	Amoebic abscess	F	Hydatid cyst
B	Ascending cholangitis	G	Portal pyaemia – appendicitis
C	Cholecystitis	H	Portal pyaemia – diverticulitis
D	Cryptogenic liver abscess	I	Portal pyaemia – peritonitis
E	Empyema of gallbladder		

Instructions: For each of the following scenarios, choose the single most likely diagnosis from the list above. Each option may be used once, more than once or not at all.

44. A 72-year-old man presents with overt sepsis. Some 25 years previously he underwent a successful hepaticojejunostomy reconstruction of an injured common bile duct at attempted laparoscopic cholecystectomy. His liver function is deranged, and peripheral blood cultures are consistent with Gram-negative bacilli.

45. A 60-year-old woman, who grew up on a farm, presents with weight loss, anorexia and right upper quadrant pain over a number of weeks. Her full blood count shows an eosinophilia.

46. A 38-year-old man presents with anorexia and weight loss over a 3-week period. He frequently works abroad, where medical attention has been difficult to obtain. One month earlier, he suffered from an episode of significant illness. He described lower abdominal pain, fevers, and pelvic irritation symptoms. These symptoms settled, but he now complains of upper abdominal pain. Ultrasound confirms two focal areas of liver abscesses.

Theme: Cholangiocarcinoma

A	CT with triple phase contrast	F	Full coagulation profile
B	Diagnostic laparoscopy	G	Magnetic resonance cholangiopancreatography
C	Duplex ultrasonography		
D	Endoscopic ultrasound and FNA	H	Percutaneous biopsy – CT guided
E	Endoscopic retrograde cholangiopancreatography (ERCP) with or without drainage	I	Proceed to radical resection
		J	Percutaneous transhepatic cholangiogram with or without drainage

Instructions: For each of the following scenarios, choose the single most likely intervention from the list above. Each option may be used once, more than once or not at all.

47. A 72-year-old man presents with a short history of painless jaundice. An ultrasound demonstrates a heterogeneous lesion around the hilum of the liver, without obvious signs of portal vein thrombosis.

48. An 80-year-old woman has been diagnosed with locally advanced cholangiocarcinoma. On imaging, it is proximal, extends into the intrahepatic biliary tree and has probable portal vein encasement. She is a frail inpatient with increasing bilirubin levels and borderline renal function. Routine chest X-ray incidentally demonstrated a sizeable diaphragmatic hernia on the left.

49. A 54-year-old man presents with painless jaundice of abrupt and recent onset. Imaging studies to date have shown a small but malignant-looking lesion just at the biliary confluence, possibly impinging on the portal vein.

Answers: SBAs

1. B Laparoscopic cholecystectomy on the next available list

Laparoscopic cholecystectomy should be performed, and no further ductal imaging is necessary (given the dimensions of the duct on ultrasound and normal blood tests). However, given that this case is representative of simple biliary colic, frequently exacerbated by pregnancy, there is no urgency for the procedure in the absence of any complications. Once a decision has been made that surgery is necessary (e.g. in unresolved cholecystitis), this should go ahead irrespective of the pregnancy. If the patient is unwell, the indications for emergency abdominal surgery in pregnancy are the same in the acute setting as for non-pregnant women (SAGES; 2011). Full counselling and support from the obstetric team is advised. Laparoscopic approaches may also be safely adopted. Given that the patient is young, and has suffered symptoms from her gallstones, it would equally be wrong to follow the option of dietary advice alone.

2. B CT of the abdomen

The most likely diagnosis here is a head of pancreas tumour with painless jaundice and systemic upset. The previous history of calculi is a red herring, but the sphincterotomy would result in a dilated duct, so that such a finding at ultrasound may be irrelevant. An ultrasound is most useful in probable benign jaundice to establish the presence of calculi and ductal dimensions, so determining whether decompression is necessary at subsequent endoscopic retrograde cholangiopancreatography. A magnetic resonance cholangiopancreatography may be a useful adjunct in this case, in terms of assessing ductal anatomy, and possible staging information. Only if the tumour is deemed resectable would an endoscopic ultrasound be carried out to fully assess nodal status. This presentation is more characteristic of locally advanced disease.

3. C Laparoscopic cholecystectomy with on-table cholangiogram

In this scenario, the patient continues to suffer pain and inflammation and she therefore needs an intervention to remove the source of the problem. The raised bilirubin and transaminase levels are likely to reflect a hepatic response to the cholecystitis. However, on-table cholangiography is prudent to exclude ductal calculi (**Figure 5.1**). If ductal stones are revealed, treatment options include ductal exploration or postoperative endoscopic retrograde cholangiopancreatography (ERCP) (if local expertise is not available). It is highly likely she will not require an ERCP, and the risks of this intervention can be safely avoided. If the patient's symptoms improve, then an MRCP prior to laparoscopic cholecystectomy without a cholangiogram would be the best option.

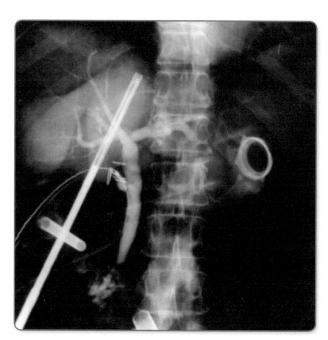

Figure 5.1 On-table cholangiogram demonstrating normal biliary anatomy.

It is well-documented that recurrent admissions with cholecystitis will continue until the problem is removed, with each episode associated with risks of jaundice/pancreatitis, and potentially, increasingly difficult procedures. A meta-analysis conducted by Lau et al. (2006) also suggests a cost benefit with early laparoscopic cholecystectomy (in terms of reduced total time in hospital and comparable morbidity profiles). These principles also apply to elderly patients, if general operative fitness is reasonable.

4. B Pylorus-preserving pancreaticoduodenectomy may be the preferred treatment option for patients with advanced disease

The standard 'Whipple's' pancreaticoduodenectomy (PPD), or the modified PPD, is being used increasingly in centres of expertise on the grounds that, in selected patients, radical resection may afford a somewhat improved quality of life with less pain than other palliative options. There is a risk that, within the projected survival timeframe postoperatively, patients may never fully regain general quality of life to benefit fully from the procedure.

Although such an approach may be adopted, it is recommended only in centres of expertise that routinely audit patients' disease extents, resections, and outcomes. Only patients deemed fit and potentially suitable for surgery based on CT should undergo more invasive staging investigations, such as endoscopic ultrasound (EUS), preoperatively. EUS may be necessary in the context of equivocal nodes on CT, as sensitivity is increased using EUS. Surgery may form a very important component of management in locally advanced disease. Palliative duodenal bypass surgery may be the safest and easiest option to afford the patient good symptomatic control with more rapid surgical recovery.

Improvements in the medical oncology management of the disease, with chemoradiation protocols based on gemcitabine and capecitabine, have afforded patients some advantages in the management of this previously hopeless disease.

5. D Men are relatively more at risk of HCC than women

Screening for hepatocellular carcinoma (HCC) is worthwhile in the at-risk population. This includes those with established cirrhosis or hepatitis C virus (HCV). In a population with no endemic hepatitis, general population screening is not justifiable. HCV is more likely to lead to HCC than hepatitis B virus (HBV). Elderly men are most at risk of malignant transformation in any pre-existing liver disorder. Primary biliary cirrhosis (more common amongst women) is relatively less associated with malignant change. α-Fetoprotein and ultrasound are the recognised screening modalities in at-risk groups. These are currently used in established cases of HBV and HCV, cirrhosis, haemochromatosis and men with alcohol-induced cirrhosis who are currently abstinent and likely to comply with treatment. CT and MRI are then used to confirm a likely diagnosis. 20–50% patients with HCC have undiagnosed cirrhosis and have therefore escaped surveillance.

6. D Previous chemotherapy administration may limit the extent of surgery offered

The surgical management of colorectal liver metastases has evolved significantly in the last decade. If lesions are resected, patients may expect a 40% chance of 5-year survival, and a second presentation with new metastases following successful resection may still be considered for surgery, dependent on the time interval and extent of liver involved already resected. After each successful resection, the patient's survival rates are restored to the same postoperative baseline, with the same perioperative morbidity profiles. Accepted UK practice follows the guidance from the American Hepato-Pancreato-Biliary Association (2006), which state that lesions should be considered resectable if the disease can be completely resected, two adjacent liver segments can be spared with adequate vascular inflow and outflow and biliary drainage, and the volume of liver remaining will be adequate. In an otherwise normal liver, this is limited to 20%, but multiple factors increase the necessary threshold, not least previous chemotherapy administration which often results in steatohepatitis. If there is concern about the extent of surgery required to resect all disease, patients may undergo a staged, two-part procedure to allow liver regeneration between operations. If adequate synthetic function is recovered, the second, curative operation may proceed. Similarly rarely, chemotherapy may also be used to downstage disease to a respectable extent. This is unique to colorectal disease. Radiofrequency ablation has a recognised side effect profile of bleeding, biliary tree injury and sepsis occurring in around 9% patients. It remains an alternative treatment for patients unfit for surgery, and may 'enhance' resectability, although it is not without risk.

7. B Severe pancreatitis is defined as organ(s) failure and/or local pancreatic complications

Objective scoring should support clinical assessment for appropriate management plans.

Option B is the correct definition of a severe attack, complemented by the presence of other unfavourable prognostic signs. In the first 24 hours, severity is best predicted by experienced clinical judgement, APACHE II score >8 and obesity, whilst at 48 hours, Glasgow Coma Score ≥3, C-reactive protein >150 mg/L and persistent organ failure are the most useful tools. APACHE III, IV and simplified acute physiology score II (SAPS II) have also been developed and used in this context, but are not specific to pancreatitis.

8. B Gallstones account for approximately 35% of cases, with approximately 15% of patients developing acute pancreatitis

Although gallstones account for 30–40% of all cases of pancreatitis, only 5% of patients with stones have a resultant episode of acute pancreatitis. Small stones and male sex are significantly associated with an increased risk of pancreatitis. More unusual aetiologies include triglyceridaemia, pancreas divisum, vascular compromise (including vasculitis), and drug-induced (furosemide, azothioprine, thiazides). The UK guidelines (Working Party BSG et al., 2005) provide not only useful treatment guides, but a comprehensive overview of aetiology and risks. Sanders and Kingsnorth (2007) have also described the epidemiological outcomes of gallstone disease in detail.

9. D Staged laparotomies with open abdominal wound management systems successfully manage pancreatic necrosis

Pancreatic necrosis and pseudocysts have a range of management options including radiology, endoscopy, surgery, and conservative management. It is recommended that necrosis of >30%, established at 1–2 weeks following presentation with pancreatitis, should have fine-needle aspiration performed for culture and sensitivity. Patients with probable sepsis and even lesser volume necrosis should have the same, prior to starting any antibiotics. The antimicrobial choice should be guided by early microbiology information. If aspiration is performed too early, the aspirate may well be sterile. Ongoing sterile necrosis, without symptoms to suggest sepsis, may be managed conservatively without adverse effects.

Septic necrosis will require surgical or radiological drainage, depending on the extent and the expertise available. Closed systems of lavage following open necrosectomy can enable ongoing lavage. A staged procedure with planned re-laparotomies, lavage and packing minimises the risk of too radical an approach at one sitting, and the risk of abdominal compartment syndrome, which may already be significant.

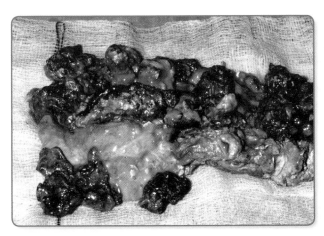

Figure 5.2 A pancreatic necrosectomy which illustrates the extent of necrosectomy that can be required to alleviate symptoms and ongoing inflammatory responses.

An example of the extent of necrosectomy can be seen in **Figure 5.2**. Depending on the size and location of a pseudocyst, they may be managed conservatively (normal if <6 cm), or via surgical (open or laparoscopic), endoscopic, or radiological means.

10. C Ongoing alcohol consumption should be primarily addressed, even in established pancreatitis

Alcohol is the most common underlying cause of chronic pancreatitis, and evidence supports addressing its ongoing use irrespective of the stage of presentation. Surgical interventions may be used in refractory cases, the most common procedures being a duodenum-preserving resection of the pancreatic head, or Frey's ductal decompression (pancreaticojejunostomy). In a selective group of patients, endoscopic decompression of the pancreatic duct was a useful pain-relieving measure in two-thirds of the population, whereas biliary decompression may be necessary to relieve associated jaundice or cholangitis. Neither dietary fat restriction nor enzyme supplementation have been shown to reduce pain, but may be helpful in relieving malabsorptive steatorrhea.

11. A Obtain a tissue diagnosis with core biopsy

This patient has had a previous high-risk breast carcinoma; despite the passage of time, the possibility of late metastatic disease always remains. In her case, the presentation was incidental to one triggered undoubtedly by symptomatic gall stones. Offering her a laparoscopic cholecystectomy may be a reasonable next step, as there are a number of therapeutic options available to her, which may give her a relatively prolonged survival. However, on discovery of this 'incidental' disease, although recurrence is the most likely cause, a tissue diagnosis is required, with the ability to perform receptor status analysis in order that therapy can be appropriately tailored. Breast cancer remains an enigma for hepatic surgery and, at present, there is no evidence advocating a resectional approach. It may well be more 'systemic' in nature at the point of recurrence than other solid tumour types, and therefore remains under oncological management.

12. A Serum chromogranin and urinary 5-hydroxyindoleacetic acid levels are useful in the diagnosis

Neuroendocrine tumours are rare and difficult to diagnose. Diagnosis is dependent on correct recognition of the hormonal symptoms in conjunction with accurate, multimodality imaging investigations, often involving nuclear medicine. It may be some time before any such neoplasia becomes symptomatic, either from pressure effects or hormonal influence. The majority of cases are sporadic, but may represent part of a multiple endocrine neoplasia syndrome, or in conjunction with neurofibromatosis-1. Serum chromogranin A is a protein produced by neural crest-derived cells, with urinary 5-hydroxyindoleacetic acid most sensitive for midgut tumours. If there is a suspicion of a broader syndrome, appropriate screening with thyroid function tests, parathyroid levels, αFP, CEA β-hCG, calcium, calcitonin and prolactin should be carried out.

13. E Vaccinations should include polyvalent pneumococcus, *Haemophilus influenzae* B and meningococcus

Depending on local transfusion practice/policy, a cross-match is non-essential prior to splenectomy. Group and save is routine with preoperative haemoglobin, and platelet count. Platelets are only required preoperatively in the context of thrombocytopaenia (often immune thrombocytopaenic purpura [ITP] is the indication for surgery). When platelets are required they should be administered immediately prior to surgical manipulation. In the emergency setting, a red cell cross match would be expected. Although vaccinations are ideally administered more than 2 weeks prior to elective surgery, failure does not preclude surgery. This is of no immediate concern in the emergency setting. In such a scenario, they should then be given more than 2 weeks postoperatively. Patients should be warned of the small but significant risk of both postoperative sepsis, and lifelong vulnerability to infections, applicable irrespective of operative indication.

14. B Laparoscopic splenectomy is a safe option in immune thrombocytopaenic purpura

Safety is well-established for a laparoscopic approach in this condition. Appropriate perioperative transfusion of platelets should be given as required, and this should be delayed until as close as possible to surgical control of the splenic vessels, so that rapid breakdown of transfused products may be avoided. The choice of laparoscopic or open approach is made on a case-by-case basis. However, this is influenced not only by surgeon expertise, but also by the degree of splenomegaly and the underlying condition. For example, massive splenomegaly in myelofibrosis requires open surgery. Increasing use of surgical technologies, staplers and haemostatis dissectors and large retrieval bags, means that the upper size limit may be stretched. Such vascular staplers may control the hilar vessels en-bloc, and precise dissection is therefore not required. Laparoscopic splenectomy has been shown to be safe and to provide comparable haematological results with a reduced rate of postoperative complications. Hence, it is increasingly the procedure of choice for normal to moderately enlarged spleens in elective patients.

15. A Beta-blockade prevents re-bleeding in a proportion, but does not reduce overall mortality

In 'left-sided' portal hypertension, caused by splenic vein thrombosis (which may then result in gastric varices and bleeding), splenectomy is curative. Current guidance recommends that only grade II or III varices are managed pharmacologically with non-selective beta-blockade using propranolol or nadolol. This was based on the findings of a meta-analysis by D'Amico et al (1999) which also demonstrated a reduced bleeding risk from 25% to 15% over a minimum 24-month follow-up period. Withdrawal of treatment may lead to a return to the original risk. Overall mortality is not reduced by treatment, but withdrawal from treatment may increase mortality. In contrast, following a bleed, beta-blockade does impact on mortality, with a meta-analysis demonstrating a 7% reduction in mortality compared with controls.

16. A A cystic duct stump leak is included in formal classification systems

There are two formal systems of bile duct injury classification: the five part Strasberg system (a stepwise classification of biliary injuries, from minor to severe, **Table 5.1**) and a separate classification system of transactional biliary injuries described by Bismuth (**Table 5.2**). The full extent of injury may not be apparent at the initial surgical event, requiring careful imaging to define them. Even a cystic duct stump leak will require drainage during the time taken to heal (ordinarily achieved by re-laparoscopy, placement of abdominal drain and then endoscopic retrograde cholangiopancreatography [ERCP] to define the injury and allow placement of a biliary stent-drain). Drainage is preferentially internal, and the abdominal drain may be removed, and repeat ERCP/removal of stent performed at an appropriate interval to allow healing. Thus, the extent of intervention for any degree of biliary injury should not be underestimated.

Table 5.1 Strasberg classification of biliary injury	
Strasberg classification	Definition
A	Leakage from the cystic duct stump or subvesical ducts
B	Occlusion of part of the biliary tree, most usually aberrant right hepatic ducts
C	As for B, but with transection instead of ligation
D	Lateral injury to the biliary tree, e.g. distal common duct, but without complete transection
E	Transactional injuries to the common hepatic duct, and more proximal (classified 1–5 as per Bismuth)

Table 5.2 Bismuth classification of biliary injury	
Bismuth classification	Definition
1	Low common hepatic duct stricture – hepatic duct stump >2 cm
2	Proximal hepatic duct stricture – hepatic duct stump <2 cm
3	Hilar stricture with no residual common hepatic duct – hepatic duct confluence intact
4	Destruction of hepatic duct confluence – right and left hepatic ducts separated
5	Involvement of aberrant right sectoral hepatic duct alone or with concomitant stricture of the common hepatic duct

17. A A ductal T-tube and a subhepatic drain offer a temporising measure before definitive management

This is the safe option and is recommended unless expert help is available from an independent surgeon competent to perform a hepaticojejunostomy (**Figure 5.3**). Carroll et al. (1998) demonstrated that 79% of injury repairs had a successful outcome when referred to experienced, independent surgeons, but only 27% were successful in the hands of the primary operator. Direct closure and placement of a T-tube may be feasible, but help should be sought from an independent surgeon whenever injury is suspected. Abdominal drains should be

Figure 5.3 Hepaticojejunostomy.

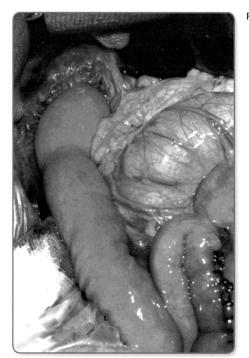

free of bile staining by 24 hours postoperatively. If there is complete transection of the duct, endoscopic retrograde cholangiopancreatography cannot aid in diagnosis, and percutaneous transheptic cholangiography may be necessary, in addition to contrast CT or magnetic resonance cholangiopancreatography.

The consequences of major biliary injury, with potential for strictures and recurrent cholangitis, liver atrophy and cirrhosis later in life cannot be emphasised enough. Optimal management must be instituted whenever major injury is suspected. Poor prognosticators are involvement of the biliary confluence, repair by the primary surgeon, or recent active inflammation.

18. B Adenomatous polyps of the gallbladder measuring <3 cm may be followed with serial ultrasounds

Gallbladder carcinoma is uncommon, notoriously presenting late, and often picked up incidentally at cholecystectomy. There are markers of underlying malignancy including a calcified, porcelain gallbladder (**Figure 5.4**). This finding indicates chronic inflammation, which is associated with an increased risk of developing cancer (overall incidence 10%). The current recommendation is for cholecystectomy, but with normal, non-urgent operative work-up. Any cause for chronic inflammation of the gallbladder represents a risk factor for subsequent malignancy and hence the presence of an enteric fistula falls within this category.

Adenomatous gallbladder polyps, present in 1% of cholecystectomy specimens, have malignant potential. The risk rises with increasing size >1cm, patient age and multiple polyps. Lesions which are smaller than 1cm may be safely followed with sequential scans, but >1cm is an indication for surgery. If malignancy is suspected, further imaging (CT/MRI) should be performed to exclude nodal disease, and appropriate operative plans made. The patient and surgeon should both be prepared for an appropriate extent of resection, depending on operative findings. Preoperative tissue diagnosis is not mandatory.

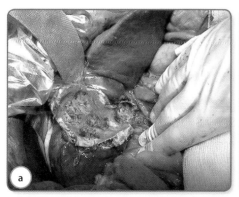 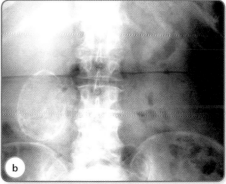

Figure 5.4 (a) Operative appearances of a porcelain gallbladder, necessitating conversion to open cholecystectomy. (b) Radiograph showing a porcelain gallbladder.

19. A 5-year survival rates of 25–40% exist for those undergoing complete, curative resections

The overall prognosis of this relatively uncommon tumour remains poor, and it is relatively chemo- and radiotherapy resistant. Palliative options are less likely to include standard cancer treatments, but are more likely to include percutaneous or surgical bypass/drainage procedures. Option D is false, in that surgical intervention may in fact be very important in this group of patients. The most important prognostic factor in patients undergoing resection is obtaining clear resection margins, associated with the 5-year survival rate quoted above. Only in tertiary specialist centres, amongst a very selective patient group, can liver transplantation be considered and it remains experimental.

Answer: EMIs

20. C Endoscopic retrograde cholangiopancreatography and sphincterotomy

This patient should undergo urgent endoscopic retrograde cholangiopancreatography and sphincterotomy followed by laparoscopic cholecystectomy. Therapeutic endoscopic retrograde cholangiopancreatography is recommended for all cases of gallstone-related pancreatitis with signs of an obstructed duct or cholangitis. This is best performed within 72 hours of onset, with sphincterotomy regardless of whether a stone is identified (**Figure 5.5**). Despite the MRCP findings, it is likely that a stone has passed, and this procedure should prevent recurrent attacks if there is a wait for surgery. Current guidelines (BSG Working Party et al., 2005) do recommend early laparoscopic cholecystectomy on

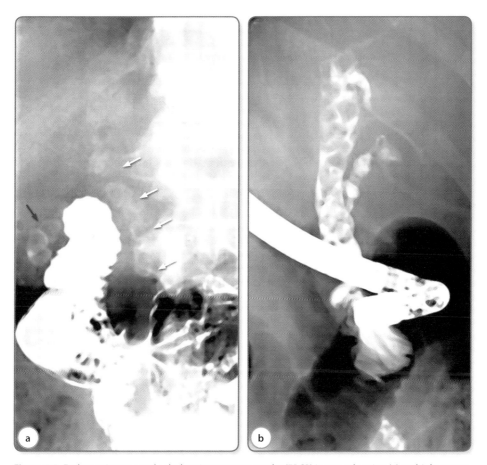

Figure 5.5 Endoscopic retrograde cholangiopancreatography (ERCP) images showing (a) multiple stones in the gall bladder (black arrow) and common bile duct (white arrows) and (b) ERCP cholangiogram showing multiple stones in the common bile duct.

the same admission, or within 2–4 weeks, in all fit patients. Proceeding straight to surgery without first clearing the duct could result in harm or recurrent attacks.

21. D Fine-needle aspiration of the pancreas then intravenous antibiotics

This patient is at risk of secondary infection within an area of pancreatic necrosis, and given his age and the severity of the disease, aggressive intervention is warranted. Current guidelines (Working Party of the British Society of Gastroenterology, 2005) suggest that antibiotics are a reasonable step in patients at risk of developing infected necrosis, his clinical risk known to correlate with necrosis in over 30% of cases. A CT-guided aspirate should be obtained first, if the collection is accessible, prior to empirical antibiotics being commenced. A Cochrane systematic review (Villatoro et al., 2006) has suggested decreased mortality in this select group of patients.

22. F Laparoscopic cholecystectomy

This patient should undergo early laparoscopic cholecystectomy in the absence of any other anatomical or obstructive concerns. This should be done in the same admission, or within a 2–4 week interval. No further biliary imaging is necessary, whether preoperative or operative. This is supported by current guidelines (recommendation level B; Jibawi and Cade, 2010).

23. I Primary sclerosing cholangitis

Although this presentation is acute with markedly deranged bilirubin and evidence of some decompensation, there is no clear immediate precipitant to suggest fulminant liver failure. This is further negated by normal liver parenchyma. Early portal hypertension and reversed flow would be in keeping with the underlying pathology of primary sclerosing cholangitis, which is associated with inflammatory bowel disease (ulcerative colitis more commonly than Crohn's disease).

24. G Head of pancreas tumour

This scenario is in keeping with a malignancy of the gallbladder or bile duct. According to Courvoisier's law, a palpable gallbladder is indicative that the underlying problem is unlikely to be due to gallstones, as they result in a shrunken, fibrotic viscus which does not easily distend. Here, the opposite is true, with overt downstream obstruction. Malignancy within the biliary tree is the most likely diagnosis, with a head of pancreas tumour the most common cause.

25. C Cholecystitis

This presentation is in keeping with acute cholecystitis, causing a secondary bilirubin rise, with raised inflammatory markers and local tissue reaction. At this patient's age, an 8 mm common bile duct is within normal limits, and the LFT picture is not particularly obstructive. This picture should settle expectantly but, should she proceed to same admission cholecystectomy, a cholangiogram [intraoperative, or magnetic resonance cholangiopancreatography (MRCP)] would be advisable unless LFTs settle completely. Around 70% of patients with symptomatic gallstones are expected to develop further symptoms or complications within 2 years after a first presentation, and so intervention is definitely recommended. An operative picture of a 'hot gallbladder', a commonly used term for an acutely inflamed gall bladder, is seen in **Figure 5.6**. Increasing numbers of surgeons are offering safe, same admission surgery following first presentation with such disease – with the increasing availability of MRCP, this is no longer dependent on 'routine' intraoperative cholangiogram. Here, a fistula is demonstrated.

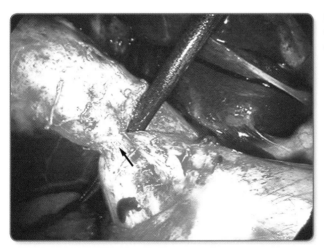

Figure 5.6 Operative picture of cholecystitis. The arrow points to a cholecyst-duodenal fistula.

26. G Type IVb

The Todani classification is shown in **Table 5.3** (Todani et al., 1977).

Table 5.3 The Todani classification	
Todani classification	**Description**
Ia	Dilatation of extrahepatic bile duct (entire)
Ib	Dilatation of extrahepatic bile duct (focal segment)
Ic	Dilatation of the common bile duct portion of extrahepatic bile duct
II	True diverticulum from extrahepatic bile duct
III	Dilatation of extrahepatic bile duct within the duodenal wall (choledochocoele)
IVa	Cysts involving both intra- and extrahepatic ducts
IVb	Multiple dilatations/cysts of extrahepatic ducts only
V	Multiple dilatations/cysts of intrahepatic ducts only

27. A Type la

See answer 26.

28. H Type V

See answer 26.

29. E Liver transplantation assessment

This patient should be assessed for transplantation, as he fulfils the criteria for abstinence, and presents with tumours which would require an extended right resection. Given the background and degree of cirrhosis, he would be unlikely to survive this. Patients with multifocal tumours generally cannot be considered suitable for resection. Hepatocellular carcinoma is the only tumour for which transplantation can be considered. It is an attractive option in that it removes both detectable and undetectable tumour nodules, and prevents the postoperative complications which are associated with portal hypertension and liver impairment.

30. G Portal venous embolisation of tumour

This patient has multiple documented foci of hepatocellular carcinoma. Although a limited right hemihepatectomy seems attractive to clear the disease, her cirrhosis is too advanced for resection to be feasible at this stage. Similarly, she is not suitable for transplantation. Portal venous embolisation is a reasonable first line treatment to attempt to shrink the tumours down. Re-consideration may then be given to right hemihepatectomy, following assessment of her response to treatment. Radiofrequency ablation would be a reasonable approach if the lesions were more scattered, thus making resection impossible.

31. I Wedge resection/segmentectomy

The literature supports re-resection for colorectal metastasis for as long as the patient remains fit. In this case, there are no contraindications to further surgery, and with an isolated tumour an anatomical segmentectomy is a reasonable approach to management. One consensus statement (American Hepato-Pancreato-biliary Association; 2006) concluded that colorectal metastases can be resected if the disease can be completely resected, and two adjacent segments can be spared with adequate vascular in-/outflow and biliary drainage, with adequate remaining future liver volume.

32. D Cyst adenoma

Cyst adenomas tend to be found in middle aged women. They may be asymptomatic or present with right upper quadrant pain/fullness, obstructive jaundice or nausea and vomiting. They may also have normal liver function tests. They may be up to 40 cm in diameter and can be unilocular or multilocular. On ultrasound the cyst contents may range from anechoic to low level echoes from blood products/mucin/proteinaceous fluid. Cyst adenomas have malignant potential and therefore should be resected.

33. C Mesenchymal hamartoma

Mesenchymal hamartoma generally present in children under the age of 2 years, with a male predominance (2:1). They tend to present with abdominal distension and respiratory distress. Imaging ranges from showing a predominantly cystic tumour, to a multiseptated cystic tumour, to a mixed solid and cystic tumour, to even a completely solid tumour. Treatment is usually resection, although cyst aspiration to facilitate surgical resection is a recognised treatment.

34. B Liver cell adenoma

Liver cell adenoma is the most frequent liver tumour of young women on the oral contraceptive pill (OCP). They may be asymptomatic and identified incidentally on imaging for another condition, present with right upper quadrant pain, or with spontaneous bleeding into the abdomen. They are most commonly in the right lobe of the liver and are often a round, well defined, pseudo-capsulated mass. On ultrasound, they can be hyper- or hypoechoic, and are hypervascular. Treatment is discontinuation of the OCP and checking α-fetoprotein (AFP) levels (large lesions may degenerate into hepatocellular carcinoma). Small lesions may be observed with imaging and AFP levels however large lesions (>5 cm) should be removed surgically in view of the potential for haemorrhage and malignant transformation.

35. F Multiple endocrine neoplasia-1 (MEN-1) syndrome

This presentation is most in keeping with a glucagonoma. This is the second most commonly involved organ within an underlying multiple endocrine neoplasia-1 (parathyroid involvement is the commonest abnormality). There is no explanation of this patient's previous need for total parathyroidectomy. However, four-gland hyperplasia (without background renal failure) would normally trigger screening investigations for an underlying disorder. Various protocols exist for screening investigations in the context of such disorders.

36. B Carcinoid syndrome

In this scenario, it is likely that the patient's appendix specimen demonstrated a carcinoid tumour on histology. Current recommendations state that if the tumour is >1 cm, or incompletely excised, a completion right hemicolectomy is necessary. This only represents the minority of cases, with tumours most commonly <1 cm, and situated at the tip (75%) or middle (15%) of the appendix. The carcinoid syndrome results when the tumour metastasises to the liver, causing hormonal release (serotonin, etc) directly into the systemic circulation. In addition to the description here, patients can also present with palpitations and lacrimation. Metastases are very rarely amenable to resection.

37. I Zollinger–Ellison syndrome

This scenario describes Zollinger–Ellison syndrome. A gastrin-secreting tumour (commonly a pancreatic endocrine tumour but with extrapancreatic tumours also included in the definition) commonly presents with epigastric pain and non-healing peptic ulcers. When the lesion is pancreatic, two-thirds of patients will have multifocal disease, and should have full functional imaging performed. This includes radioimmunoassay of serum gastrin levels and measurement of gastric acid secretion, along with somatostatin receptor scintigraphy. CT and endoscopic ultrasound may also be combined to provide full anatomical information. The diagnosis does raise the possibility of a multiple endocrine neoplasia syndrome. Management should address both elements of (i) treatment of gastric hypersecretion and (ii) excision of the tumour(s).

38. B Endoscopic stenting of common bile duct (CBD) only

This young patient may well have resectable disease but until full staging information can be completed, it would be preferable to relieve his jaundice. Pancreatic duct stenting would only be considered when the lesion is not resectable, for now all that is required is biliary drainage, which can be attained via endoscopic retrograde cholangiopancreatography (ERCP) and stent insertion. A plastic stent should be used, as metal stents may render the disease more difficult to resect in the future. Cytology may also be obtained with ERCP, however false negative rates are high, and this should not negate appropriately aggressive surgery if the appropriate and informed consent is obtained. There is little evidence to support relief of jaundice prior to definitive surgery but, if surgery is to be delayed by more than 10 days it is recommended that drainage is achieved and surgery delayed to allow the jaundice to resolve.

39. E Open bypass procedure: gastrojejunostomy

This woman has locally advanced, surgically unresectable disease. Her systemic symptoms would suggest a degree of advancement in the disease process. However, she also has a degree of gastric outlet obstruction, and so unless her general fitness precludes surgery, a palliative bypass procedure should be offered. A straightforward gastrojejunostomy can be constructed to bypass the mechanical blockage, leaving the biliary anatomy intact. Various bypass procedures can be considered depending on the exact presentation of symptoms. Without surgery, patients with this type of presentation have at least a 20% risk of complete gastric outlet obstruction, supported by trial data in one series (Lillemoe et al., 1999).

40. H Referral for chemoradiation treatment

At 80 years of age with locally advanced disease (but no symptomatic issues), this man should be considered for chemoradiation. Portal vein involvement is another surgical contraindication. Chemoradiation was initially utilised for neoadjuvant and adjuvant purposes in patients with palliative treatment intent. However, increasingly encouraging results from gemcitabine-based regimens, with concurrently favourable side effect profiles, mean that this option may provide a survival advantage for patients without the side effect profiles of older chemotherapy regimens. It may also have improved efficacy and quality of life when compared to overly radical surgery (which would be inappropriate). In younger, fitter patients, there is also a chance that such a regimen, begun with palliative intent, may render such a disease resectable. The response should be assessed carefully.

41. B Budd–Chiari syndrome

This is a rare condition resulting from occlusion of the hepatic veins, and presenting with pain, ascites, and either acute fulminant or chronic liver failure. The caudate lobe tends to hypertrophy, and the compensation this provides is life-preserving. Haematological assessment is required. It should be noted that there is a documented association with oral contraceptive pill (OCP) use, although OCP use is also associated with liver adenoma. The treatment of the acute condition normally comprises transjugular intrahepatic portosystemic shunt decompression, which restores hepatic venous outflow across at least one channel. If the patient then develops fulminant liver failure, emergency transplantation is the only option. High success rates are reported with shunts, but the patients will require long-term anticoagulation.

42. F Portal vein thrombosis

Portal pyaemia with secondary thrombosis is a rare but recognised complication of any intra-abdominal sepsis (most commonly diverticulitis and appendicitis). Extensive mesenteric thrombosis can result and patients may then present with gut infarction. Diagnosis may be made on Doppler ultrasound examination or CT angiogram. Active treatment normally requires full anticoagulation. A case series is reported by Sheen et al. (2000). A very extensive example, with thrombus throughout the portal vasculature, can be seen in the CT in **Figure 5.7**. This patient presented with abrupt onset, severe generalised abdominal pain – worryingly, no precipitant reason was identified for his underlying portal vein thrombosis, so he was heparinised and endovascular decompression was carried out.

43. E Myelofibrosis

This case represents a form of 'presinusoidal' portal hypertension, whereby increased splenic flow caused by massive splenomegaly produces a hypertensive portal circulation. Although the diabetes may lead to a suspicion of haemochromatosis, there is no hepatomegaly or evidence of cirrhosis and no other stigmata are mentioned. Portal hypertension occurs in approximately 10% of patients with myelofibrosis, and following splenectomy the condition can be reversed.

44. B Ascending cholangitis

Although this patient seems to have achieved a good result from his biliary reconstruction, such patients remain at risk of ascending infections in the interim and

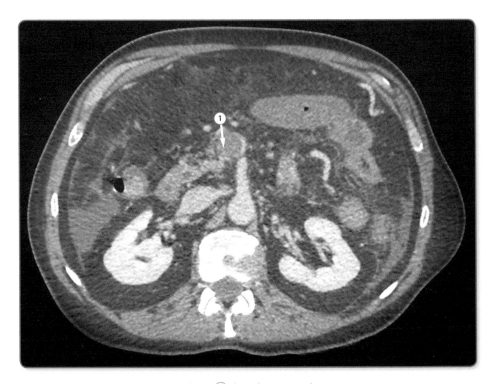

Figure 5.7 Extensive portal vein thrombosis. ① Thrombus in portal vein.

the bacteriology result here is typical of such a scenario. There are also limited reports of secondary carcinomas at the site of reconstruction. No prophylaxis is recommended routinely for such patients, unless they require stenting with ongoing episodes of stent-cholangitis. As a first episode, this man should be treated appropriately with intravenous antibiotics and any liver abscess should be drained percutaneously.

45. F Hydatid cyst

Echinococcus infection is a zoonosis that can lead to liver infections, sometimes many years after the initial exposure to dog or sheep sources. Most infections are latent for many years, only presenting when complications occur. Secondary infections occur in around 10% of cases with abnormal liver function and eosinophilia. Serology may aid the diagnosis, but radiology is also useful, typically demonstrating a calcified cystic wall, and septa within the cyst cavity. Percutaneous drainage is to be avoided because of the risk of both dissemination and anaphylaxis. Surgery is usually required.

46. G Portal pyaemia – appendicitis

It is increasingly common that presentations of liver abscess are secondary to more common intra-abdominal pathology; the history here is typical for appendicitis, which seems to have settled conservatively, but not without sequelae. The patient in question is a little too young to suspect diverticulitis, but this is an important differential and, along with colonic neoplasm should be considered in older patients with histories of altered bowel habits. Other sources of haematogenous spread leading to liver abscess include bacterial endocarditis and pneumonia – non-gastrointestinal sources account for 10–20%. Nonetheless, biliary sepsis remains by far the most common underlying cause of liver abscess.

47. A CT with triple phase contrast

In the scenario, the cholangiocarcinoma is a new diagnosis, but ultrasound is insufficient to inform on resectability and likely staging. Cross-sectional imaging, most commonly CT, remains essential in evaluating such patients in terms of level of obstruction, vascular involvement and liver atrophy. It does tend to underestimate the extent of the tumour within the bile duct proximally. This may not be the primary determinant of resectability, necessitating magnetic resonance cholangiopancreatography and duplex examination. These additional procedures may also be necessary if the CT provides no obvious contraindications.

48. J Percutaneous transheptic cholangiogram with or without drainage

In this scenario, the tumour is non-resectable, particularly given the clinical condition of the patient. Adequate investigations appear to have been carried out to define this and she should proceed with the best palliative option available. Conversely, it is important in potentially curative cases to proceed with all necessary non-invasive investigations prior to contemplating drainage interventions. This reduces the risk of patient morbidity and infectious complications. Here, a drainage procedure is required, and would be most easily achieved via a percutaneous, transhepatic approach. It may also be impossible to pass an endoscope through her pylorus, if the stomach is intrathoracic.

49. C Duplex ultrasonography

CT angiography is traditionally used to examine portal vein/hepatic vessel involvement in biliary tumours. It is specifically used to examine cholangiocarcinoma at the hilum, but duplex ultrasound has been shown to be superior (albeit with operator dependent factors). Respective sensitivity and specificity for ultrasound versus CT were 93 and 99% versus 90 and 99% respectively. It is also useful for precisely delineating the level of the tumour within the bile duct. In this scenario, the rate limiting step will be portal vein involvement, so this investigation is critical.

Chapter 6

Transplantation surgery

Questions: SBAs

For each question, select the single best answer from the five options listed.

1. A 22-year-old man is taken to intensive care following a road traffic accident, where his condition deteriorates. He is a card-carrying organ donor.

   Which of the following conditions is not a prerequisite for the confirmation of brainstem death?

   A Absent corneal reflex
   B Absent vestibulo-ocular reflexes
   C Apnoeic coma
   D Absence of respiratory movements when $Paco_2$ >6.65 mmHg
   E Absence of response to supraorbital pressure

2. A 68-year-old woman receives a renal transplant from her twin sister.

   What is the most common surgical complication?

   A Haemorrhage
   B Lymphocoele
   C Renal artery stenosis
   D Renal artery thrombosis
   E Urinary leak/fistula

3. A 58-year-old man with interstitial nephritis receives a cadaveric renal transplant. Ten days later he remains dependent upon haemodialysis. An ultrasound identifies a 15 × 12 cm perigraft collection and a urinary catheter is inserted.

   What is the most appropriate management?

   A Aspiration of the fluid and injection of sclerosant
   B Aspiration of the fluid for biochemical analysis
   C Conservative management
   D Digital subtraction angiography to localise haemorrhage source
   E Surgical re-exploration

4. A 42-year-old man receives a cadaveric renal transplantation and is commenced on antirejection treatment, which includes cyclosporin.

   What is the most common side effect of cyclosporin?

   A   Alopecia
   B   Hepatotoxicity
   C   Nephrotoxicity
   D   Pancreatitis
   E   Pancytopaenia

5. Which of the following options mediates hyperacute renal transplant rejection?

   A   Complement
   B   Immunoglobin E (IgE)
   C   Natural killer cells
   D   T-helper lymphocytes
   E   T-suppressor lymphocytes

6. A 42-year-old man receives a cadaveric renal transplantation and begins antirejection treatment which includes azathioprine.

   What is the most common side effect of azathioprine?

   A   Alopecia
   B   Hepatotoxicity
   C   Nephrotoxicity
   D   Pancreatitis
   E   Pancytopaenia

7. A 57-year-old man with diabetes consults his physician asking about the possibility of a pancreas transplant from his twin sister.

   Which of the following is not an indication for pancreatic organ transplant?

   A   Insulin-dependent diabetes with end-stage renal failure
   B   Insulin-dependent diabetes with unawareness of hypoglycaemia
   C   Insulin-dependent diabetes with uncontrolled ketoacidosis
   D   Non-insulin dependent diabetes with end-stage renal failure
   E   Non-insulin dependent diabetes with uncontrolled ketoacidosis

8. A 65-year-old man with diabetes develops end-stage renal failure.

   With which of the following criteria may he still be placed on the waiting list for a renal transplant?

   A   Antiglomerular basement membrane disease with circulating antibody
   B   Immunosuppression predicted to cause life-threatening complications
   C   Predicted risk of graft loss >30% at 1 year
   D   Predicted patient survival of <5 years
   E   Unable to comply with standard immunosuppressant therapy

9. A 54-year-old woman with diabetes is considering her options for pancreatic transplantation.

   Which of the following is not a benefit of pancreatic islet cell transplantation over pancreatic solid organ transplantation?

   A It can be performed under local anaesthesia
   B There is a higher rate of insulin independence
   C There is less need for immunosuppression
   D There is lower morbidity
   E There is lower mortality

10. Which of the following statements does not describe living-donor liver transplantation?

   A 55–70% of the liver can be removed from a healthy living donor
   B Liver donors commonly require blood transfusion
   C The donor remnant should regain 100% function by about 6 weeks
   D There is a 0.5–1.0% chance of death for the donor
   E There is a complication rate of up to 10% for the donor

11. A 54-year-old man with marked jaundice attends the transplant unit after hearing about celebrities who have successfully received a liver transplant.

   Which of the following diagnoses is liver transplantation not indicated for?

   A α1-antitrypsin deficiency
   B Cholangiocarcinoma
   C Hepatocellular carcinoma
   D Primary biliary cirrhosis
   E Primary sclerosing cholangitis

12. A 58-year-old man with insulin-dependent diabetes and end-stage renal failure has poor hypoglycaemic awareness and is considered for a pancreas transplant.

   What is the most appropriate treatment?

   A Pancreas-after-kidney transplantation
   B Pancreatic islet transplantation
   C Pancreas transplant alone
   D Solitary kidney transplantation
   E Simultaneous pancreas and kidney transplantation

13. A 55-year-old woman has had a functioning renal transplant for 6 months. She has now developed a tremor in addition to headache, nausea and diarrhoea. On examination, she has bleeding gums and biochemistry reveals abnormal renal function.

Which antirejection drug is the most likely cause of these side effects?

A Azathioprine
B Cyclosporin
C Mycophenolate mofetil
D Prednisolone
E Tacrolimus

14. A 48-year-old man with insulin-dependent diabetes is considered for a pancreatic islet transplantation.

Which of the following is not an indication for pancreatic islet transplantation in those with insulin-dependent diabetes?

A Insulin-dependent diabetes with end-stage renal failure
B Inadequate autonomic symptoms
C Metabolic lability
D Secondary complications
E Unawareness of hypoglycaemia

15. A 54-year-old woman receives a cadaveric renal transplantation.

Which of the following statements does not describe delayed graft function (DGF) in her situation?

A Acute transplant rejection is associated with DGF
B Cold ischaemia time is associated with DGF
C DGF alongside early acute rejection has a 5-year graft survival rate of 70%
D DGF has a more deleterious effect on graft survival than human leukocyte antigen (HLA) mismatch
E DGF is associated with diminished kidney allograft survival

16. Which of the following statements describes graft survival following renal transplantation?

A Complete (0/6) human leukocyte antigen (HLA) mismatch transplants can be used
B One-year graft survival has decreased over the last decade, particularly from deceased donors
C One-year graft survival is lower from HLA mismatched (1–5/6) living donors than 6/6 matched deceased donors
D One-year graft survival is lower in complete HLA matched (6/6) than mismatched (1–5/6) donors
E One-year graft survival is lower in living donor compared to deceased donor transplants

17. A 58-year-old man who died from a cerebrovascular accident was found to be carrying an organ donor card. He qualifies to donate a kidney as an 'expanded criteria donor'.

Which of the following options in his medical history would result in reduced graft quality?

A   Creatinine >10 mg/L (>76 µmol/L)
B   End-stage renal failure
C   Insulin-dependent diabetes
D   Previous coronary artery bypass graft
E   Previous squamous cell carcinoma of skin

18. A 27-year-old woman with short gut syndrome is being considered for intestinal transplantation.

When considering the indications for intestinal transplantation, which of the following statements are false?

A   Irreversible intestinal failure with life-threatening complication(s) of parenteral nutrition
B   Extensive severe mesenteric arterial disease requiring intervention
C   Metastatic malignant disease requiring extensive evisceration
D   Localised neuroendocrine tumour requiring extensive evisceration
E   Extensive desmoid disease requiring extensive evisceration

Questions: EMIs

Theme: Antirejection medication

A   Alemtuzumab
B   Antilymphocyte globulin
C   Antithymocyte globulin
D   Basiliximab
E   Cyclosporin
F   Daclizumab

G   Mycophenolic acid
H   Mycophenolate mofetil
I   Prednisolone
J   Rituximab
K   Sirolimus
L   Tacrolimus

Instructions: For each of the following descriptions, choose the single appropriate medication from the list above. Each option may be used once, more than once or not at all.

19. A chimeric mouse-human monoclonal antibody to the α-chain (CD25) of the T-cell's IL-2 receptor. Used in renal transplant.

20. Administered prior to stem cell transplant to kill T cells and lower the risk of graft-versus-host disease (GVHD).

21. A macrolide antibiotic that binds to FK506-binding protein 12 (FKBP12) to form a complex that inhibits calcineurin. Used for organ rejection prophylaxis in liver, kidney, and heart transplants.

Theme: Components of the immunological response

A   Antigen presenting cells
B   CD4 surface protein
C   CD8 surface protein
D   Complement
E   Cytokines
F   Dendritic cells
G   Immunoglobin (IgE)
H   Major histocompatibility complex

I   Macrophages
J   Natural killer cells
K   T-cell receptor
L   T-helper lymphocytes
M   T-suppressor lymphocytes (regulatory T-cells)
N   Toll-like receptor

Instructions: For each of the following descriptions, choose the single most likely component from the list above. Each option may be used once, more than once or not at all.

22. Cells which recognise glycolipid antigen and once activated, perform functions of both T-helper and cytotoxic T cells (cytokine production and release of cytolytic molecules). They are therefore able to recognise and eliminate tumour cells.

23. These antigen presenting cells express both surface proteins CD4 and CD8, and are critical for cell mediated immunity.

24. T-cell receptor co-receptor which binds specifically to class I major histocompatibility complex.

Theme: Transplant types

A   Heterotopic allograft
B   Heterotopic autograft
C   Heterotopic isograft
D   Heterotopic xenograft
E   Orthotopic allograft

F   Orthotopic autograft
G   Orthotopic isograft
H   Orthotopic xenograft
I   Syngeneic heterotopic graft
J   Tandem transplant

Instructions: For each of the following scenarios, choose the single most appropriate transplant from the list above. Each option may be used once, more than once or not at all.

25. A 45-year-old man with hepatocellular carcinoma receives a liver transplant from his identical twin who died in a road traffic accident that day.

26. A 55-year-old man with insulin-dependent diabetes and end-stage renal failure has a simultaneous pancreas and kidney transplant from a random deceased extended criteria donor.

27. A 68-year-old man receives a kidney transplant from his elder brother.

Theme: Transplant variations

A   Corneal transplant
B   Donation after brainstem death donor (DBD) heart transplant
C   DBD liver transplant
D   DBD renal transplant
E   Donation after cardiac death donor (DCD) liver transplant

F   DCD renal transplant
G   Extended criteria renal transplant
H   Living donor liver transplant
I   Living donor renal transplant
J   Pancreatic islet transplant
K   Pancreas alone solid organ transplant

Instructions: For each of the following scenarios, choose the single most appropriate transplant from the list above. Each option may be used once, more than once or not at all.

28. The transplant which is most commonly affected by vascular thrombosis.

29. A 58-year-man develops intraparenchymal liver tract bleeding 2 days after his transplant procedure.

30. The solid organ transplant with the highest 1-year postprocedural graft survival.

Theme: Donor choice

A   Brain-death donor, blood-group A, Rhesus –ve (HLA 5/6)

B   Brain-death donor, blood-group AB, Rhesus +ve (HLA 5/6)

C   Brain-death donor, blood-group AB, Rhesus +ve (HLA 5/6)

D   Brain-death donor, blood-group O, Rhesus +ve (HLA 1/6)

E   Cardiac-death donor, blood-group A, Rhesus –ve (HLA 5/6)

F   Cardiac-death donor, blood-group AB, Rhesus +ve (HLA 1/6)

G   Cardiac-death donor, blood-group B, Rhesus +ve (HLA 6/6)

H   Cardiac-death donor, blood-group O, Rhesus +ve (HLA 6/6)

I   Living donor, blood-group A, Rhesus +ve (HLA 5/6)

J   Living donor, blood-group A, Rhesus –ve (HLA 4/6)

K   Living donor, blood-group AB, Rhesus +ve (HLA 2/6)

Instructions: For each of the following scenarios, choose the single most appropriate donor from the list above. Each option may be used once, more than once or not at all.

31. A 66-year-old woman (blood group AB negative) requires a simultaneous pancreas and kidney transplant.

32. A 47-year-old man (blood group B negative) requires a kidney transplant.

33. A 35-year-old man (blood group A negative) requires a kidney transplant.

Theme: Post-transplant complications

A   Acute rejection
B   Cytomegalovirus infection
C   Hepatic artery thrombosis
D   Hepatitis
E   Lymphocoele
F   Obstructive uropathy
G   Pancreatitis
H   Peritransplant haematoma

I   Pneumonia
J   Renal artery occlusion/stenosis
K   Renal vein thrombosis
L   Transplant venous thrombosis
M   Urinary tract infection
N   Urinoma
O   Wound infection

Instructions: For each of the following scenarios, choose the single most likely complication from the list above. Each option may be used once, more than once or not at all.

34. A 62-year-old man has had an orthotopic liver transplant 10 days ago. He is now profoundly jaundiced and is vomiting gastric contents. He is pyrexial with a temperature of 38.6°C and feels generally 'unwell'.

35. A 49-year-old woman is 6 days post-pancreatic alone transplant with pancreaticoduodenocystostomy. She has haematuria and is tender in her right iliac fossa. She has raised blood glucose. Serum amylase is normal but there is a low urinary amylase. There is no evidence of an immunological component.

36. A 39-year-old woman develops the infection that is most common following an allogenic renal transplant.

Theme: Malignancy following solid organ transplant

A	Bladder cancer	H	Malignant melanoma
B	Breast cancer	I	Mouth, tongue and lip cancer
C	Cervical/vulval cancer	J	Neuroblastoma
D	Colorectal cancer	K	Non-Hodgkin's lymphoma
E	Kaposi's sarcoma	L	Non-melanomatous skin cancer
F	Kidney/ureteric malignancy	M	Prostate cancer
G	Lung cancer	N	Thyroid cancer

Instructions: For each of the following scenarios, choose the single most likely malignancy from the list above. Each option may be used once, more than once or not at all.

37. A 47-year-old man has a renal allograft from a matched donor. He is diagnosed with Epstein–Barr virus infection and later develops a related malignancy.

38. A 62-year-old woman with a well-functioning renal allograft develops the most common post-transplant de novo malignancy.

39. A 49-year-old Indian man with a previous renal transplant is diagnosed with human herpesvirus-8. He later develops cutaneous lesions with visceral involvement.

Answers: SBAs

1. D Absence of respiratory movements when Pa_{CO_2} >6.65 mmHg

In the UK, rules for the diagnosis of brainstem death were published in 1976 and have only been slightly modified since.

The preconditions for consideration of brain death are:

- The patient should be comatose, unresponsive and ventilated because of irreversible brain damage of known aetiology
- There should be no sedating medication
- Hypothermia as the cause of unconsciousness must be excluded
- Reversible circulatory, metabolic and endocrine disturbances must be excluded
- Reversible causes of apnoea (e.g. muscle relaxants or cervical cord injury) must be excluded

Once these preconditions are satisfied, brainstem death can be tested for by two doctors together, on two separate occasions with an unspecified interval between. Both of these doctors must have been registered for at least 5 years, neither should be members of the transplant team, and at least one must be a consultant.

The definitive criteria are:

- Fixed unresponsive pupils
- Absent corneal reflex
- Absent oculovestibular/caloric reflexes (no eye movements following the injection of at least 50 mL of cold water into each ear)
- No response to supraorbital pressure
- No cough/gag reflex to bronchial/pharyngeal stimulation
- No respiratory effort in response to hypercapnia; this requires preoxygenation prior to disconnection from the ventilator, followed by a period of approximately 5 minutes to allow elevation of the Pa_{CO_2} to at least 6.0 kPa, or 6.5 kPa in those with CO_2 retention.

2. B Lymphocoele

Allogenic renal transplant is a successful procedure which carries a low complication rate. However, in addition to rejection and delayed graft function, there are also a variety of surgical complications which can cause significant morbidity. Any of the three anastomoses (renal artery, renal vein, or ureter) can be involved and wound infections and fluid collections also feature.

Renal artery stenosis occurs in up to 10% but thrombosis is rare (<1%). Renal vein problems occur in a similar percentage of patients and when examined overall, vascular complications account for 5–10% of all postoperative complications. Urinary leak occurs in up to 10% and may lead to urinoma or fistula. Renal artery or vein complications and urinary leaks will all require surgical (or radiological) intervention.

Postoperative haemorrhage is uncommon and occurs in 1% of patients. Lymphocoele is the most common postoperative complication and can occur in up to 50% of patients.

3. B Aspiration of the fluid for biochemical analysis

In this patient's situation, conservative management is inappropriate because of the renal dysfunction. Initial management of any fluid collections associated with graft dysfunction should include inserting a urinary catheter to decompress the bladder. Approximately 1–10% of patients develop post-transplant perirenal fluid collections. These collections can be lymphocoeles, urinomas, seromas or haematomas.

In the immediate postoperative period, any identified collection could be due to a haematoma, urinoma or seroma. Collections that develop in the weeks to months following the procedure are more likely to be a lymphocele or rarely an abscess. The patient in this scenario requires confirmation of the cause of his fluid collection and a urinoma can be diagnosed by performing fluid aspiration and biochemical assessment. A higher creatinine level in the aspirate fluid compared with its serum concentration differentiates a urine leak from a seroma or lymphocoele. If there is diagnostic uncertainty, a MAG3 radioisotope renal scan can be performed which would confirm the diagnosis of a urinoma if radionuclide is retained in the collection. A positive diagnosis of urinoma can be followed by further imaging studies (such as a percutaneous nephrostogram) to identify the site of the leak.

Urinomas occur early in the postoperative course, most commonly because of leakage at the ureteroneocystostomy (which may be secondary to necrosis of the distal ureter). Small urinary leaks can be controlled by bladder drainage alone, but if this fails to resolve then intervention is required. Antegrade or retrograde double-J stenting of the ureter may be sufficient although the collection may also require formal percutaneous drainage. If these minimally invasive techniques fail to manage the urinary leak, an open surgical approach and reconstruction may be necessary.

4. C Nephrotoxicity

Cyclosporin is a calcineurin inhibitor which inhibits the production of cytokines (such as interleukin-2 and interferon-γ) resulting in inhibition of T-lymphocyte activation. Since its introduction to the routine immunosuppression in the postrenal transplant antirejection regime, cyclosporine has dramatically improved long- and short-term graft outcomes.

The main limitation in the use of cyclosporine is its main side effect – nephrotoxicity. Other side effects also include hirsutism, gingival hyperplasia, tremor and hypertension.

5. A Complement

Hyperacute rejection occurs within the first 24 hours after transplantation and is characterised by graft thrombosis and haemorrhage occurring within minutes to hours after the graft is implanted. This is a type III hypersensitivity reaction whereby the immune complex is mediated by the complement system.

It occurs due to pre-existing host antibodies that are directed against antigens present in the graft endothelium. The complement system is activated by antigen recognition resulting in an increase in neutrophils with endothelial and platelet activation. This results in a hypercoagulable state with inflammation, scarring and ischaemia.

Acute rejection is a type II hypersensitivity reaction mediated by T-cells, and chronic rejection is a type IV hypersensitivity reaction mediated by both humoral and cellular mechanisms.

6. E Pancytopaenia

Azathioprine (AZA) is a precursor of 6-mercaptopurine which inhibits purine (adenine and guanine) synthesis and thereby blocks the cell cycle. The most common serious side effect of AZA therapy is pancytopaenia, and in particular leukopaenia, which makes patients particularly prone to infection. Other less common side effects include alopecia and <1% may develop pancreatitis or hepatotoxicity.

Nephrotoxicity is associated with calcineurin inhibitors such as cyclosporin and to a lesser extent tacrolimus. Mycophenolate mofetil (MMF) acts via a similar mechanism to AZA, but is associated with less bone marrow suppression and, in conjunction with lower rejection rates, is preferred if the higher cost can be justified.

7. E Non-insulin dependent diabetes with uncontrolled ketoacidosis

In most cases, pancreas organ transplantation is performed as a simultaneous pancreas and kidney (SPK) transplant in patients with problematic type 1 diabetes with end-stage renal disease (ESRD). With changing patient demographics and an increasing proportion of type 2 diabetes, approximately 6% of SPK recipients are people with diabetes.

In type 1 diabetes with ESRD, there are three transplant options:

- Solitary kidney transplant alone
- Simultaneous pancreas and kidney transplant
- Pancreas-after-kidney transplant

If there is no renal dysfunction, a pancreas alone transplantation may be performed. In type 1 diabetes, severe hypoglycaemic events and hypoglycaemic unawareness are the most common indication for pancreatic transplant. Hyperglycaemia, ketoacidosis which requires medical attention and clinical or emotional problems with exogenous insulin resulting in incapacitation, as well as complications despite insulin therapy, are all consider indications for pancreatic transplant.

8. C Predicted risk of graft loss >30% at 1 year

The UK transplant guidelines (Kasiske et al., 2001) list several contraindications for renal transplantation. Absolute contraindications include:

- Predicted patient survival of <5 years
- Malignant disease not amenable to curative treatment, or remission for > 5 years
- HIV infection
- Severe cardiovascular disease
- Predicted risk of graft loss >50% at 1 year
- Anti-glomerular basement membrane (anti-GBM) antibody disease with circulating antibody
- Inability to comply with immunosuppressant therapy

Immunosuppression can cause life-threatening complications, owing to:

- Unresolved chronic bacterial infection
- Persistent viral infection

9. B There is a higher rate of insulin independence

Islet cell transplantation is a radiological procedure which can be performed under local anaesthesia with minimal risk. Purified islets are isolated from the digested pancreas (normally from more than one donor) prior to percutaneous transhepatic injection into the portal vein. Through immunological tolerance, it is hoped that in the future islet transplantation could be performed without the need for immunosuppression. Although it is a far safer procedure than a solid organ transplant, the success of islet transplantation is limited by its measured procedural success. Approximately 14% of diabetic patients are independent of insulin at 1 year post islet transplantation, compared to 82% of patients following a vascularised pancreas transplant.

10. B Liver donors commonly require blood transfusion

In living donor liver transplantation, a section of liver is removed from a healthy living person and is transplanted into a recipient, following the removal of the diseased liver. Normally 55–70% of the liver (normally the right lobe) can be removed from the healthy donor and within 4–6 weeks it should regenerate to almost 100% function. Full volumetric size is normally reached shortly afterwards. The transplanted part should achieve full function and the appropriate size in a slightly longer period of time.

The risk of complications in the donor is approximately 10%, and these commonly include biliary fistula, gastric stasis and infection. Very few donors will require blood transfusion, either during or after surgery. The risk of death for the donor ranges from 0 to 1% depending upon the case series.

11. B Cholangiocarcinoma

Patients are considered for liver transplantation if they have:

- Fulminant hepatic failure
- A serious complication of liver disease
- Cirrhosis (with complications such as hepatic encephalopathy or ascites)
- Hepatocellular carcinoma
- Hepatorenal syndrome
- Bleeding due to portal hypertension

Cholangiocarcinoma (CCA) is an absolute contraindication to liver transplantation (**Table 6.1**) in most centres, because of the poor transplant outcome in studies performed in the 1980s and 1990s. In 1987 the European transplant registry reported a 0% survival at 5 years post-liver transplantation for CCA. Later studies have also reported poor 5-year survival rates ranging from 10–38%.

Table 6.1 Contraindications to liver transplantation	
Absolute	**Relative**
AIDS	Age >70 years
Cholangiocarcinoma	Extrahepatic sepsis
Severe cardiopulmonary disease	Hepatitis B
Synchronous malignancy	HIV
	Ongoing alcohol or substance misuse
	Portal vein thrombosis
	Psychiatric illness
	Pulmonary hypertension

12. E Simultaneous pancreas and kidney transplantation

Solitary kidney transplantation (SKT) does not incorporate any form of pancreas transplantation because it is a 'single kidney transplant'. Pancreatic islet transplantation is contraindicated in patients with end-stage renal failure (ESRF). Because this patient has ESRF, he should not have a 'pancreas transplant alone (PTA)' because this will not address his renal failure. The two main options for this patient are a SPK or a pancreas-after-kidney (PAK) transplant. SPK is performed more commonly than PAK as it is a combined procedure and the long-term graft results are superior. The international pancreas transplant registry (25,000 cases) has shown that at 1-year post-transplant, pancreas graft survival was 86% in SPK transplants, compared to 80% in PAK grafts and 78% in PTA (Organ Procurement Transplantation Network, 2012).

13. B Cyclosporin

This patient is demonstrating some fairly non-specific side effects (headache, nausea and diarrhoea). However, the symptoms of tremor and bleeding gums (due to gingival hypertrophy) and the finding of abnormal renal function, are highly suggestive of the side effect profile of cyclosporin therapy. Other common side effects of cyclosporin include hirsutism and transient hepatotoxicity. Nephrotoxicity is the most serious side effect and requires in-vivo monitoring of cyclosporin levels. Treatment with cyclosporin is limited to 9 months to reduce the chance of long-term nephrotoxicity.

14. A Insulin-dependent diabetes with end-stage renal failure

The main indication for islet transplantation is type 1 diabetes with labile disease, resulting in either reduced awareness of hypoglycaemia or other autonomic symptoms. Other indications include metabolic lability (or instability) with two or more episodes of severe hypoglycaemia, or hospital admissions with ketoacidosis during the previous 12 months. Secondary complications, such as autonomic neuropathy, are also an indication for islet transplantation.

A creatinine clearance less than 80 mL/min is a contraindication to islet cell transplantation (**Table 6.2**). Such a patient would fare better with a solid organ pancreas transplant, either as a simultaneous pancreas and kidney transplant or as a pancreas-after-kidney transplant.

Table 6.2 Contraindications to pancreatic islet transplantation
Contraindications to pancreatic islet transplantation
Age <18 years
Body weight >75 kg
Body mass index >26 kg/m^2 (female), >27 kg/m^2 (male)
Insulin requirement of >0.7 IU/kg/day or >50 IU per day (whichever is less)
Positive C-peptide response (≥0.2 ng/mL) to glucose tolerance testing
Creatinine clearance <80 ml/min/1.73 m^2
Positive pregnancy test
Active infection including hepatitis C, hepatitis B, HIV, or tuberculosis
Invasive aspergillus infection during the previous 12 months
History of malignancy (except for treated basal cell carcinoma or small cell carcinoma)
Active alcohol or substance abuse
History of non-adherence to prescribed medical regimens
Unstable psychiatric disorder
Inability to provide informed consent
Severe coexisting cardiac disease
Abnormal liver function tests
Gallstones or liver haemangioma
Coagulopathy or requirement for long-term anticoagulant therapy
Active peptic ulcer disease
Severe gastrointestinal disorders interfering with ability to absorb oral medication

15. C DGF alongside early acute rejection has a 5-year graft survival rate of 70%

Acute transplant rejection occurs more frequently in grafts with delayed graft function (DGF). Ojo al. (1997) analysed the USA renal data system records of 37,216 primary cadaveric renal transplants between 1985 and 1992. They demonstrated acute transplant rejection in 37% of patients with DGF compared to 20% in grafts without.

Similarly, Shoskes and Cecka (1998) analysed 27,000 cadaveric donor renal transplants reported to the UNOS Scientific Renal Transplant Registry between 1994 and 1997, demonstrating acute rejection in 8% of patients without DGF and in 25% of patients with DGF.

The deleterious impact of delayed function is comparatively more severe than that of poor HLA matching. There is an approximate 23% increase in the risk of DGF for every 6 hours of cold ischaemia. DGF appears to be independently predictive of 5-year graft loss. DGF in conjunction with early acute rejection results in only a 5-year graft survival rate of 35%.

16. A Complete (0/6) HLA mismatch transplants can be used

For all transplants a living donor kidney is better than a deceased donor kidney. This is regardless of human leukocyte antigen (HLA) matching and at all time points. It is considered that a zero match living donor organ has better survival than a perfectly matched deceased donor organ. The closer the HLA match is, the longer the graft survival and this effect increases over time. Graft survival rates are best for a perfect (six out of six) match, followed by HLA matching of one to five antigens, with the poorest graft survival rates for an unmatched graft (**Figure 6.1**).

There have been modest improvements in graft survival rates over the last 10 years with the greatest improvements in the deceased donation group.

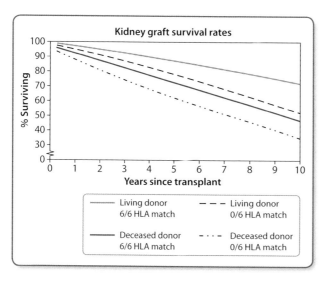

Figure 6.1 Kidney graft survival rates.

17. B End-stage renal failure

Expanded (or extended) criteria donors (ECD) have been considered for renal transplants because of the shortage of available 'ideal' donors and the increasing demand for organs. Medical factors which make allografts less than ideal include increasing age, hypertension, diabetes and increased risk of transmitting infection or malignancy. Cause of death as a cerebrovascular accident (CVA) and abnormal renal morphology or function can also contribute to reduced graft quality.

The organ procurement and transplantation network (OPTN) have subsequently recommended that all donors above the age of 60 years, and any donors aged 50–59 years with at least two out of three medical criteria (CVA as cause of death, hypertension, creatinine >15 mg/L), are classified as expanded ECD.

18. C Reflux pancreatitis

The indications for intestinal transplantation are:

1. Irreversible intestinal failure with:
   - life-threatening complications of parenteral nutrition [progressive intestinal failure-associated liver disease (IFALD) or non-IFALD despite all remediable actions, severe sepsis, exhaustion of central venous access]
   - very poor quality of life thought to be reversible by transplantation
2. Patients with indications for extensive surgery involving partial or complete evisceration:
   - extensive desmoid disease
   - extensive severe mesenteric arterial disease requiring intervention
   - localised neuroendocrine tumours
3. Patients requiring transplantation of other organs where exclusion of simultaneous intestinal transplantation would adversely affect patient survival

The absolute contraindications are:

1. Metastatic malignant disease
2. Systemic disease with poor prognosis
3. Severe neurological diseases with progressive impairment

The relative contraindications are:

1. Active generalised sepsis or severe systemic infection
2. Requirement for ventilatory support
3. Neurological diseases with permanent sequelae
4. Insufficient venous access
5. Systemic disease with a life expectancy <5 years
6. Neoplastic disease with an uncertain prognosis
7. Psychosis unlikely to respond to full treatment and result in nonadherence
8. Patients unlikely to adequately comply with post-small intestinal transplant treatment
9. Age >60 years

Answer: EMIs

19. D Basiliximab

Basiliximab is a chimeric mouse-human monoclonal antibody to the α-chain (CD25) of the T-cell IL-2 receptor. It is used to prevent rejection in renal transplantation in the immediate postoperative period. It has also been used off licence in cardiac and liver transplantation, and in graft versus host disease.

20. B Antilymphocyte globulin

Antilymphocyte globulin (ALG) is an immunosuppressant agent used in the treatment of acute rejection in organ transplantation, as well as lowering the incidence of chronic graft versus host disease after stem-cell transplantation. It is a polyclonal antibody that acts on T-cell surface antigens and depletes CD4 lymphocytes.

21. L Tacrolimus

Tacrolimus is a macrolide antibiotic that binds to FK506-binding protein 12 (FKBP12) to form a complex that inhibits calcineurin. Transplant patients generally remain on lifelong calcineurin inhibitors even if all other immunosuppressant drugs are withdrawn.

22. J Natural killer cells

Natural killer (NK) cells are innate immune system lymphocytes, which are involved in the early defence against foreign cells and cells undergoing infection or tumour transformation. NK cell activation is initiated upon interaction with the antigen presented on cells targeted for destruction. These NK cells express a wide variety of cell surface receptors which can trigger cytolytic cascades and cytokine secretion, leading to targeted cell death.

23. F Dendritic cells

Dendritic cells are vital to the presentation of peptides and proteins to T and B lymphocytes and are important antigen presenting cells (APCs). They induce T cell responses resulting in cell-mediated immunity. CD4 is expressed on monocytes, macrophages, dendritic cells and T-helper lymphocytes, whereas CD8 is expressed on dendritic cells and cytotoxic T cells. CD4 and CD8 therefore play important roles in major histocompatibility complexes (MHC), as antigens expressed on the cell surface which activate T-helper cells which has important effects on the regulation of the immune system.

24. C CD8 surface protein

CD4 and CD8 precursor cells differentiate to become mature CD4+ and CD8+ T cells. These express T-cell receptors which recognise any foreign antigens associated with the major histocompatibility complex (MHC) class I (CD8+) or class II (CD4+) molecules. The role of the MHC is to display antigens so that they can be recognised by T lymphocytes.

The CD8 molecules on CD8+ T cells bind to a site found only on class I histocompatibility molecules.

The CD4 molecules on CD4+ T cells bind to a site found only on class II histocompatibility molecules.

As CD8 can only bind to a receptor site on class I histocompatibility molecules, CD8+ T cells are therefore only able to respond to antigens presented by class I molecules. Similarly, CD4 molecules expressed on the surface of CD4+ T cells are able to bind to cells presenting antigen in class II molecules (but not in class I). All cell types can present antigens with class I molecules, whereas only certain cells (those able to take up antigen from extracellular fluid) can present antigens with class II molecules.

25. G Orthotopic isograft

'Orthotopic' and 'heterotopic' refer to the site where a transplant is performed. An orthotopic transplant is grafted to the normal anatomical site in the donor. An example of this is the liver which is normally transplanted to the same site following the removal of the diseased liver. An isograft transplant is taken from a donor to a genetically identical recipient, such as occurs between identical twins. Another term for 'genetically identical' is 'syngeneic'.

26. A Heterotopic allograft

A heterotopic transplant is taken from a different site from the diseased recipient organ. The recipient organ can therefore be left in situ. Kidney and pancreas organ transplants are always heterotopic. An allograft is a transplant from one genetically different member of a species to another. Most renal transplants are therefore allografts.

27. A Heterotopic allograft

As in Question 26, it is a heterotopic allograft.

With regards to organ transplantation:

- An **allograft** describes a transplant from one genetically different member of a species to another. Most renal transplants are therefore allografts.
- An **autograft** (or autogenic graft) is when tissue is transplanted from one site to another on the same patient (e.g. a skin graft or flap reconstruction).

- An **isograft** describes the transplantation from a donor to a genetically identical recipient, such as occurs between identical twins. Another term for 'genetically identical' is 'syngeneic'.
- A **xenograft** is a transplant from a different species.

Orthotopic and heterotopic refer to the site where a transplant is performed.

- **Orthotopic** is a transplant to the normal anatomical site in the donor. An example of this is the liver which is normally transplanted to the same site following the removal of the diseased liver.
- **Heterotopic** is transplantation to a different site from the diseased recipient organ. The recipient organ can therefore be left in-situ. Kidney and pancreas organ transplants are always heterotopic.

A tandem transplant is a technique used in patients receiving stem cell therapy, whereby they receive two sequential courses of high-dose chemotherapy with their transplant.

28. K Pancreas alone solid organ transplant

Complications following solid organ pancreas transplant have steadily decreased over the last 10–15 years. Surgical complications remain common and are 2–3 times more common, than following renal transplantation. The pancreas is a low flow organ and is therefore particularly prone to graft thrombosis. Approximately 5–8% of pancreatic organ transplants will develop venous or arterial thrombosis which will ultimately lead to technical failure of the graft.

29. J Pancreatic islet transplant

Pancreatic islet transplantation is performed via the percutaneous transhepatic route. This avoids the need for general anaesthetic and many of the complications of open surgery which contribute to the higher morbidity and mortality associated with pancreatic organ transplant.

Life-threatening acute blood tests have been reported in islet recipients following this approach, although serious complications can be reduced by successfully obliterating the intrahepatic portal catheter track.

Table 6.3 Graft survival			
Graft type	**3 months (%)**	**1 year (%)**	**3 years (%)**
Kidney (living donor)	94.3	91.4	86.2
Kidney (deceased donor)	87.2	81.0	72.7
Liver	77.7	69.9	62.2
Pancreas	83.6	73.5	67.1
Heart	91.5	81.5	73.4
Lung	86.8	70.4	52.6
Heart and Lung	81.9	61.9	49.6

30. I Living donor renal transplant

Currently, 1-year patient and graft survival rates exceed 90% in most transplant centres. Good comparisons of survival of different transplant types can be seen from the 1997 UNOS report of 97,587 solid organ transplants in the USA. They showed 1-year graft survival of 91.4% for living donor renal transplants, which was higher than deceased renal donor, liver and heart transplants in that order (**Table 6.3**).

31. I Living donor, blood-group A, Rhesus +ve (HLA 5/6)

For all transplants, the preferred donor option is a live donor, followed by a donation after brainstem death donor (DBD), and lastly a donation after cardiac death (DCD) donor. Rhesus status has absolutely no bearing on the decision as it will not affect the transplant.

A patient with blood group 'AB' is the universal recipient and can receive a transplant from a donor with any blood group. Therefore, the living donor with the best human leukocyte antigen (HLA) match (5/6) should be used.

32. D Brain-death donor, blood-group O, Rhesus +ve (HLA 1/6)

A patient with blood group 'B' can only receive a transplant from a donor with blood group 'B' or the universal donor group 'O'. Of the three remaining options none are from a living donor and two (options G and H) are from a DCD donor. The DBD donor therefore represents the best transplant option.

33. I Living donor, blood-group A, Rhesus +ve (HLA 5/6)

A patient with blood group 'A' can only receive a transplant from a donor with blood group 'A' or the universal donor group 'O' (**Table 6.4**). Either of the two group A living donors should be considered, and the human leukocyte antigen 5/6 match donor should be chosen over the 4/6 match donor.

34. A Acute rejection

Acute liver rejection is when the recipient immune system attacks the donor liver. There is often a degree of 'biological' upset in the immune system following a transplant which may result in altered liver function tests. This needs to be carefully distinguished from a 'clinically relevant' rejection.

Significant rejection occurs in up to 40% of cases and normally in the first 7–10 days after the transplant. Symptoms of acute liver rejection may include non-specific features such as a high temperature, vomiting or diarrhoea. Features of obstructive jaundice (icteric skin/sclera), pale stools, dark urine and pruritus may also be prominent. The Banff schema is an accurate and functional system used to grade acute liver allograft rejection. It uses a global assessment to classify liver disease from indeterminate, through mild and moderate to severe rejection. It also examines portal, bile duct and venous inflammation. This system allows for comparison of data between units and for assessing prognostic significance.

35. L Transplant venous thrombosis

A raised blood glucose and low urinary amylase is suggestive of pancreatic graft failure. After rejection, vascular thrombosis is the second most common cause of pancreatic transplant failure. The pancreas is a low flow organ which is predisposed to the development of thrombosis. Additional risk factors include donor obesity and atherosclerotic disease, and a prolonged organ preservation time.

Pancreatic failure due to arterial or venous thrombosis classically occurs in the first 7 days post-transplant and may present with:

- Increased serum blood glucose
- Increased insulin requirement
- Decreased urinary amylase

If the cause is venous thrombosis (in which case it is likely to be a cuff of the portal vein, anastomosed to the common or external iliac vein, which has thrombosed) there may be symptoms of:

- Haematuria (if a pancreaticoduodenocystostomy is present)
- Graft swelling and tenderness

Bladder drainage should be attempted to reduce pressure effects and an ultrasound should be performed to determine if the transplant has adequate perfusion and venous drainage. If there is not, the patient should be explored and a graft pancreatectomy performed.

The diagnosis should not be confused with pancreatitis, which is commonly caused by ischaemic preservation injury or bladder reflux. It would classically present with graft tenderness, fever and hyperamylasaemia.

36. M Urinary tract infection

Urinary tract infection (UTI) is the most common infection in the transplant recipient, with an incidence of more than 30% in the first 3 months following renal transplantation. The presentation varies from asymptomatic patients with bacteriuria, to pyuria, pyelonephritis and even septicaemia. Unfortunately, graft dysfunction may also be a presenting feature.

An efficient host defence against infection is reliant upon a functionally intact kidney. Consequently it is unsurprising that UTIs are more common in patients with a donor ureter implanted into their own bladder. The standard urinary pathogens are commonly responsible (*E. coli*, *Proteus* species, *Klebsiella* species, *P. aeruginosa*), but because of the transplant recipient's immunosuppressed state, opportunistic infections (e.g. by *Pneumocystis carinii*, *Listeria*, and *Nocardia*) have also been documented.

37. K Non-Hodgkin's lymphoma

Epstein–Barr virus (EBV) is a double stranded DNA virus of the herpes virus family. It is associated with a range of malignancies, including post-transplant lymphoproliferative disorder (PTLD), Hodgkin's and non-Hodgkin's lymphoma (NHL), gastric carcinoma and leiomyosarcoma. EBV infection is frequently associated with lymphoma and 98% of cases with PTLD are associated with latent EBV infection. Pretransplant EBV serostatus has been shown to be significantly associated with an increased risk of NHL in renal transplant recipients ($p < 0.001$).

38. L Non-melanomatous skin cancer

Non-melanomatous skin cancers occur very commonly in patients following organ transplantation. The aetiology is multifactorial (as for the general population) where the same risk factors (fair complexion, blue eyes, male sex, increased age, human papilloma virus (HPV) infection and UV exposure) apply. The actual prevalence of non-melanomatous skin cancer reaches 40–75% by 20 years after transplantation. Immune suppression is probably the dominant factor accounting for the increased risk of skin cancer in transplant patients. Infection with HPV may also play a role as 90% of allograft recipients are affected by this known cofactor for skin cancer development. Squamous cell carcinoma (SCC) in particular occurs in transplant patients with an incidence of 65–100 times that of the general population. In the normal population SCC is outnumbered by basal cell carcinoma (BCC) at a ratio of 4:1. However in immunosuppressed individuals SCC occurs 2–4 times more frequently than BCC.

39. E Kaposi's sarcoma

Kaposi's sarcoma presents as single (or multiple) lesions on mucosal surfaces, affecting the skin, lungs, gastrointestinal tract and lymphoid tissue. It has a complex aetiology and is poorly understood. Development of characteristic lesions requires infection with human herpes virus type 8 (HHV-8) in susceptible immunosuppressed individuals. The majority of cases of Kaposi's occur in Mediterranean, Jewish, Arabic, Caribbean or African ethnic groups and the incidence is up to 500 times higher in transplant recipients, compared to the normal population.

HHV-8 infection itself is not associated with severe illness, although there may be a transient lymphadenopathy, diarrhoea, vague fatigue or skin rash when patients are seroconverting. The development of Kaposi's is suspected to be due to reactivation of HHV-8. Fortunately, viral reactivation does not always lead to development of the disease. This has been shown in the United States where the prevalence of Kaposi's sarcoma in transplant patients was 0.5%, compared to the estimated 20% rate of HHV-8 infection.

Chapter 7

Upper gastrointestinal surgery

Questions: SBAs

For each question, select the single best answer from the five options listed.

1. What is the major disadvantage of vagal-sparing oesophagectomy?

   A It is unsuitable for benign oesophageal conditions
   B It is only suitable for advanced oesophageal tumours
   C Lymphadenectomy is completely omitted
   D The left gastric artery is not preserved
   E The vagal nerves are not preserved

2. Which of the following statements best describes early oesophageal cancer?

   A Distinction between squamous and adenocarcinomas are not required
   B Early oesophageal squamous cell carcinomas are common in the Western world
   C It excludes pT1 lesions
   D It excludes high-grade intraepithelial neoplasia
   E The chances of a cure are excellent

3. A 36-year-old woman is undergoing assessment for gastro-oesophageal reflux.

   Which of the following are true?

   A Metoclopramide enhances lower oesophageal sphincter contraction
   B Smoking enhances lower oesophageal sphincter contraction
   C pH is measured 10 cm above the lower oesophageal sphincter
   D During pH monitoring the percentage of time when the pH monitoring is <3.5 is recorded
   E A DeMeester score of ≥12 indicates reflux

4. Which of the following statements best describes endoscopic therapy?

   A Argon plasma and laser ablation can be used in patients with oesophagopulmonary fistulae
   B Argon plasma and laser ablation should only be used alongside other treatment modalities
   C Circumferential mucosal resection has a high risk of stricture formation
   D Endoscopic mucosal resection should not be considered alone for local lesions
   E Endoscopic therapies are not appropriate for use in recurrent disease

5. A 66-year-old man has just been diagnosed with Barrett's disease.

    Which of the following statements best describes Barrett's disease?

    A   Columnar mucosa is replaced by squamous mucosa
    B   Endoscopic mucosal resection and ablative therapy is appropriate treatment
    C   It is a congenital condition
    D   It is found in 5–10% of patients undergoing upper gastrointestinal endoscopy
    E   No surveillance is required for Barrett's disease

6. A 64-year-old man is found to have low-grade dysplasia on biopsy of the lower
    oesophagus.

    What is the most appropriate management?

    A   An 8–12 week course of proton pump inhibitors (PPIs) then extensive re-biopsy
    B   A 6-month course of PPI then extensive re-biopsy
    C   Nothing else required
    D   Oesophagectomy
    E   Repeat upper gastrointestinal endoscopy in 1 year

7. A 59-year-old woman has been undergoing 6-monthly upper gastrointestinal
    endoscopic surveillance having previously been found to have low-grade dysplasia
    in her oesophagus. Two consecutive examinations have shown disease regression.

    What is the most appropriate management?

    A   Continue 6-monthly surveillance for a further 2 years
    B   Increase surveillance interval to an annual basis
    C   Increase surveillance interval to every 2–3 years
    D   Increase surveillance to 5-yearly
    E   Stop further surveillance and continue proton pump inhibitors

8. A 48-year-old woman is diagnosed on oesophageal biopsies to have loss of
    ganglion cells in the myenteric plexus.

    What is the most likely diagnosis?

    A   Achalasia
    B   Barrett's disease
    C   Oesophageal cancer
    D   Pulsion diverticulum
    E   Sclerosis

9. A 44-year-old man undergoes upper gastrointestinal endoscopy and biopsies are
    reported by two gastrointestinal pathologists as being 'indefinite for dysplasia.'
    Following treatment with proton pump inhibitors and repeat endoscopy and
    biopsies 6 months later, histology reveals no definite evidence of dysplasia.

    What is the most appropriate management?

    A   Continue 6-monthly surveillance
    B   No further surveillance

C   Repeat endoscopy and biopsies
D   Routine surveillance every 2–3 years
E   Surveillance with a 2-monthly endoscopy

10. A 67-year-old man is found to have dysplasia on biopsy of the oesophagus during a recent endoscopy.

Which of the following statements best describes the endoscopic surveillance and biopsy protocol for such patients?

A   All four quadrants of the oesophagus are biopsied at 2 cm intervals
B   No more than 10 biopsies should be taken
C   No such protocol exists
D   Samples should only be taken from areas where high grade dysplasia was diagnosed previously
E   The oesophagus is biopsied randomly

11. Which of the following statements best describes the management of gastric cancer?

A   Endoscopic resection is appropriate for all T1 tumours
B   Endoscopic mucosal resection is a superior technique compared to endoscopic submucosal dissection in the management of superficial gastric mucosal lesions
C   For stage III gastric cancer a subtotal gastrectomy may be carried out if a macroscopic proximal margin of 5 cm can be achieved between the tumour and the gastroesophageal junction
D   D1 resection involves removal of the perigastric lymph nodes and those along the left gastric artery
E   D2 lymph node resection has been conclusively shown worldwide to improve cancer related outcomes

12. Which of the following statements best describes brachytherapy?

A   It can only be given once in the treatment of oesophageal cancer
B   It requires a general anaesthetic and an inpatient hospital stay
C   It usually involves the use of iridium-192
D   No randomised control trials have assessed its use in oesophageal cancer
E   This is given systemically

13. A 42-year-old man is diagnosed with gastric polyps.

Which of the following statements is correct?

A   Gastric polyps usually present with bleeding
B   The most common types of benign epithelial gastric polyps are fibroma, lipoma and hyperplastic polyps
C   Fundic gland polyps are associated with atrophic gastritis
D   Adenomatous polyps are associated with *Helicobacter pylori*
E   Most hyperplastic polyps will regress with *Helicobacter pylori* eradication therapy

14. A 55-year-old man suffers from dysphagia and is diagnosed with achalasia.

    Which of the following statements best describes achalasia?

    A   Botox has no role in the treatment
    B   Cardiomyotomy is no longer the operation of choice
    C   Forceful dilatation of the oesophagus with a balloon can produce excellent results
    D   Oesophagectomy is the operation of choice
    E   Reassurance is all that is required

15. A 72-year-old woman is found at have a solitary diverticulum in her oesophagus.

    Which of the following statements best describes oesophageal diverticulum?

    A   Achalasia does not lead to diverticulae
    B   Pulsion diverticulae are most common in the distal oesophagus
    C   Pulsion diverticulae most commonly arise from the anterolateral wall of the oesophagus
    D   Pulsion diverticulae only occur in the distal oesophagus
    E   Traction diverticulae are more common than pulsion diverticulae

16. A 64-year-old woman is diagnosed with a peptic ulceration. She has no past medical history and has not been on any medication. At endoscopy she has an ulcer proximally near the gastroesophageal junction.

    Which type of gastric ulcer does she have?

    A   Type I
    B   Type II
    C   Type III
    D   Type IV
    E   Type V

17. A 55-year-old man with no previous medical history presents as emergency with haematemesis. An upper gastrointestinal (GI) endoscopy is performed which shows blood in the upper GI tract and a visible clot in the base of an ulcer. He is resuscitated and his pulse falls to normal levels after an admission systolic pressure of 90 mmHg.

    What is the Rockall score for this patient?

    A   4
    B   5
    C   6
    D   7
    E   8

18. A 45-year-old man presents with abdominal pain, nausea and vomiting and peripheral oedema. Endoscopy is carried out and he is diagnosed with Ménétrier's disease.

Which of the following statements is false?

A   Giant rugal folds of the stomach are a feature on fluoroscopy and CT imaging
B   The antrum of the stomach is usually spared
C   Ménétrier's disease is a premalignant condition with 10% risk of malignancy per year
D   Cetuximab is first line treatment
E   Gastrectomy is always required

19. A 42-year-old man presents with chest pain and shock after an episode of severe vomiting.

What is the most likely diagnosis?

A   Aspiration pneumonia
B   Boerhaave's syndrome
C   Gastroenteritis
D   Mallory–Weiss tear
E   Myocardial infarction

20. What is the cause of Chagas' syndrome?

A   *Bacillus stearothermophilus*
B   Firmicutes
C   *Pseudomonas aeruginosa*
D   *Thermodesulfobacteria*
E   *Trypanosoma cruzi*

Questions: EMIs

Theme: Gastric lymph node stations

A	Coeliac nodes	G	Lesser curvature nodes
B	Diaphragmatic nodes	H	Middle colic nodes
C	Hepatoduodenal ligament nodes	I	Paraoesophageal nodes
D	Infrapyloric nodes	J	Posterior pancreas nodes
E	Left gastric artery nodes	K	Root of mesentery nodes
F	Left gastroepiploic nodes	L	Splenic hilum

Instructions: For each of the following descriptions, choose the single most likely lymph node group from the list above. Each option may be used once, more than once or not at all.

21. Station 10.

22. Station 3.

23. Station 15.

24. Station 9.

25. Station 14.

26. Station 7.

Theme: Oesophageal emergencies

A	Black oesophagus syndrome	G	Perforation post-photodynamic therapy
B	Blunt trauma	H	Pyloric stenosis
C	Boerhaave's syndrome	I	Second degree caustic burn
D	First degree caustic burn	J	Stent placement
E	Foreign body ingestion	K	Third degree caustic burn
F	Perforation postdilatation for achalasia	L	Zollinger–Ellison syndrome

Instructions: For each of the following descriptions, choose the single most likely diagnosis from the list above. Each option may be used once, more than once or not at all.

27. A 56-year-old man presents with a single, longitudinal tear of the lower oesophagus in the left posterolateral position.

28. A 76-year-old woman, who is acutely unwell, is found at endoscopy to have acute oesophageal necrosis which ends sharply at the oesophagogastric junction.

29. The diagnosis with the highest percentage risk of iatrogenic oesophageal perforation through instrumentation.

30. A 29-year-old man ingests a caustic substance and is found on endoscopy to have hyperaemia only with no mucosal loss and mild oedema.

31. A 41-year-old woman ingests a caustic substance and is found at endoscopy to have severe bleeding and oedema of the mucosa with deep ulceration.

32. A 37-year-old woman ingests a caustic substance and is found at endoscopy to have mucosal blistering and exudate with bleeding and oedema.

Theme: Motility disorders of the oesophagus

A   Dermatomyositis
B   Diffuse oesophageal spasm
C   Diverticulum
D   Hypertensive lower oesophageal
    sphincter spasm
E   Nutcracker oesophagus
F   Non-specific oesophageal motor
    disorders

G   Primary achalasia
H   Polyarteritis nodosa
I   Polymyositis
J   Rheumatoid disease
K   Secondary achalasia
L   Systemic sclerosis

Instructions: For each of the following descriptions, choose the single most likely diagnosis from the list above. Each option may be used once, more than once or not at all.

33. A 34-year-old man presents with cutaneous appearances of skin thickening and oedema.

34. A 54-year-old man is found to have high amplitude contractions with normal peristalsis during oesophageal manometry studies.

35. A 43-year-old man with a chronic infection of *Trypanosoma cruzi.*

36. The diagnosis that is due to progressive loss of ganglion cells in the myenteric plexus of unknown cause.

37. A 56-year-old man is found to have an abnormality in his oesophagus which can be congenital or acquired, can occur anywhere in the oesophagus and can lead to perforation or neoplastic change.

38. A 69-year-old woman is undergoing oesophageal manometry and is found to have two non-peristaltic contractions in a series of 10 swallows.

Theme: Gastric cancer

A	Chemotherapy	G	Radiotherapy
B	D1 lymphadenectomy	H	Stenting
C	D2 lymphadenectomy	I	Subtotal gastrectomy
D	Gastrojejunostomy	J	Total gastrectomy
E	No treatment	K	Total gastrectomy with en-bloc distal pancreaticosplenectomy
F	Oesophagectomy and proximal gastrectomy	L	Splenectomy

Instructions: For each of the following scenarios, choose the single most appropriate treatment from the list above. Each option may be used once, more than once or not at all.

39. A 66-year-old man, who is otherwise well, is confirmed to have a proximal third gastric cancer with no evidence of metastases on staging investigations.

40. A 70-year-old man with hypertension is confirmed on histology to have an early distal third gastric cancer with no evidence of metastases on staging investigations.

41. A 55-year-old woman, who is fit and well, is found to have a locally advanced gastric cancer with direct invasion of the tail of the pancreas. Staging reveals no distant disease in the liver or the lungs.

42. A 67-year-old man presents with dysphagia, having previously been diagnosed with advanced distal oesophageal cancer with liver and lung metastases.

43. A 78-year-old man is found at operation to have an inoperable advanced distal gastric tumour causing symptoms of gastric outlet obstruction.

44. A 75-year-old woman is deemed unfit for surgery and chemotherapy, but staging has shown she has localised proximal oesophageal carcinoma.

Theme: Treatment options in gastric and oesophageal cancer

A   Brachytherapy
B   Capecitabine, cisplatin and trastuzumab
C   Cisplatin only
D   Etoposide, doxorubicin and cisplatin (EAP) regimen
E   Epirubicin, cisplatin and continuous-infusion 5-fluorouracil (ECF) regimen
F   Etoposide, l-leucovorin and fluorouracil (ELF) regimen
G   Epirubicin, oxaliplatin and capecitabine (EOX) regimen
H   External beam radiotherapy
I   Fluorouracil, doxorubicin and methotrexate (FAMTX) regimen
J   Fluorouracil and cisplatin (FUP) regimen
K   External bean radiotherapy, paclitaxel and carboplatin
L   Taxane only

Instructions: For each of the following descriptions, choose the single most appropriate treatment from the list above. Each option may be used once, more than once or not at all.

45. This treatment causes renal toxicity and requires prehydration and inpatient admission for higher doses.

46. Gemcitabine and irinotecan are examples of this group of drugs.

47. A 78-year-old man undergoes treatment for oesophageal cancer which involves the use of a high dose radioactive source being placed down the oesophagus in proximity to the tumour.

48. A 68-year-old man has a gastric adenocarcinoma (T2, N0, M0). In the perioperative period he is offered chemotherapy.

49. A 70-year-old woman is diagnosed with metastatic gastric adenocarcinoma. Immunohistochemical staining reveals the tumour to be human epidermal growth factor receptor 2 positive.

50. A 58-year-old man is diagnosed with oesophageal adenocarcinoma (T3, N0, M0). The tumour is potentially resectable. Pre-operatively, what treatment should he receive?

Answers: SBAs

1. C Lymphadenectomy is completely omitted

Vagal-sparing oesophagectomy is only indicated for pT1a and high-grade intraepithelial neoplasia lesions as lymphadenectomy is not part of the procedure. It is not therefore indicated as suitable treatment for advanced oesophageal cancers. The surgery is performed via an upper abdominal incision and also through a neck incision. It requires the use of a stripper to part the oesophagus from the plexus. As previously stated, no abdominal lymphadenectomy is undertaken so staging of lesion with lymph nodes is not carried out. During the operation the left gastric artery is not sacrificed.

2. E The chances of a cure are excellent

Early oesophageal cancers include pT1 lesions and high-grade intraepithelial neoplasia. The expected outcomes can be very favourable if appropriate treatment is undertaken, and therefore it is imperative that the distinction is made between squamous cell cancers and adenocarcinomas so that treatment can be targeted to the underlying pathology. Squamous cell cancers are more radiosensitive than adenocarcinomas.

3. A Metoclopramide enhances lower oesophageal sphincter contraction

Smoking, alcohol and caffeine reduce lower oesophageal sphincter contraction.

During pH monitoring the sensor is placed 5 cm above the lower oesophageal sphincter. Reflux is said to occur with the pH is <4. The percentage of time when the pH is <4 is recorded, as well as the percentage of time when the pH is <4 when upright and supine, the number reflux episodes, the number of reflux episodes >5 minutes duration, and the duration of the longest reflux episode. The DeMeester score is calculated from this information. A score of >14.7 indicates reflux.

4. C Circumferential mucosal resection has a high risk of stricture formation

Endoscopic mucosal therapy is a choice between ablative and endomucosal resection. Guidance suggests that ablative therapies such as argon and laser treatment should only be used alone or in combination as part of a clinical trial (Manner et al. 2007). However, it is noted that circumferential mucosal resection has a high risk of stricture formation and patients must be warned of this potential complication before they embark on such therapy.

5. B Endoscopic mucosal resection and ablative therapy is appropriate treatment

Barrett's disease is an acquired condition, not a congenital one, which has been demonstrated to affect up to 15–20% of people undergoing upper gastrointestinal endoscopy and who also report to have chronic gastrointestinal reflux-type symptoms. The histological findings, which confirm the diagnosis of Barrett's oesophagus, are squamous cells that are replaced by columnar mucosa in the lower oesophagus. Treatment of Barrett's can comprise endoscopic mucosal resection or ablation therapy depending of the grade of dysplasia or depth of the abnormality identified.

6. A 8–12 week course of proton pump inhibitors (PPIs) then extensive re-biopsy

The current guidelines (Barr and Shepherd; 2005) recommend that two specialist gastrointestinal pathologists must confirm the diagnosis of dysplasia on a specimen and if low-grade dysplasia is confirmed a 8–12 week course of PPI should be commenced, followed by a re-evaluation which includes multiple biopsies of the area. Therefore, this patient should be commenced on a PPI for 8–12 weeks. If the low-grade dysplasia is still apparent after undergoing this treatment but remains stable, then surveillance of the area should remain on a 6-monthly basis.

7. C Increase surveillance interval to every 2–3 years

The current guidelines (Barr and Shepherd; 2005) suggest that this 59-year-old woman can have the surveillance of her low-grade dysplasia increased to 2–3-yearly as she has had two negative upper gastrointestinal endoscopies.

8. A Achalasia

This is a classical histological finding of primary achalasia. It is due to progressive loss of ganglion cells in the myenteric plexus which results in the findings at manometry of a lower oesophageal sphincter which does not fully relax on swallowing and a oesphagus which does not show signs of peristalsis. The patient will likely complain of dysphagia and this is due to impaired motility of the oesophagus and decreased lower oesophageal relaxation. Barrett's disease results in changes of squamous cells to columnar cells at the distal oesophagus.

9. D Routine surveillance every 2–3 years

This 44-year-old patient's biopsies were found to be suspicious for dysplasia and the patient then underwent a course of proton pump inhibitors (PPIs) and then repeat endoscopy and multiple biopsies after 6 months. The British Society for Gastroenterologists recommends that patients who have undergone clinical follow-up in the form of endoscopy and multiple biopsies after treatment with a PPI and who have had clear examinations can return to routine surveillance, which is what should be recommended for this patient.

10. A All four quadrants of the oesophagus are biopsied at 2 cm intervals

The British Society of Gastroenterology guidelines (Barr and Shepherd; 2005) recommend that when a patient is confirmed to have dysplasia, the oesophagus should undergo biopsies of all four quadrants at 2 cm intervals. Other areas to be biopsied include the areas which had been found to have dysplasia previously and in areas where the appearance of the mucosa gives concern of an underlying abnormality.

11. C For stage III gastric cancer a subtotal gastrectomy may be carried out if a macroscopic proximal margin of 5 cm can be achieved between the tumour and the gastroesophageal junction

Endoscopic resection can be utilised in the treatment of very early gastric cancers (T1a) but only if they are confined to the mucosa, well-differentiated, ≤2 cm and non-ulcerated. Endoscopic mucosal resection is acceptable for lesions smaller than 10–15 mm with a very low probability of advanced histology (Paris 0–IIa). However, European Society of Gastrointestinal Endoscopy guidelines (Pimentel-Nunes et al, 2015) recommend endoscopic submucosal dissection as the treatment of choice for most gastric superficial neoplastic lesions.

For stage IB–III gastric cancer, radical gastrectomy the appropriate treatment. Subtotal gastrectomy is undertaken only if a proximal margin of 5 cm can be achieved between the tumour and the gastroesophageal junction. For diffuse cancers, a margin of 8 cm is advocated. Otherwise, a total gastrectomy is required.

D1 resection implies the removal of the perigastric lymph nodes. D2 is removal of perigastric lymph nodes as well as those along the left gastric, common hepatic and splenic arteries and the coeliac axis.

D2 resection has been shown to give superior outcomes in Asian countries when compared to D1 resection. However, this has not been conclusively shown in Western countries. Dutch (Bonenkamp et al, 1995 and Bonenkamp et al, 1999), British (Cuschieri et al, 1999 and Cuschieri et al, 1996) and Italian trials (Degiuli et al, 1998 and Degiuli et al, 2004) failed to demonstrate any initial survival advantage with D2 resection, although the Italian studies suggested a trend towards a benefit in disease-specific survival for patients with T2–T4 lymph node-positive cancers treated with D2 resection. Long-term follow-up from the Dutch trials demonstrated fewer locoregional recurrences and gastric cancer-related deaths with D2 resection; however, this was offset slightly by an increase in postoperative mortality and morbidity.

12. C It usually involves the use of iridium-192

Studies have suggested that brachytherapy is a good treatment for the palliation of symptoms in oesophageal cancer, where this type of therapy has been compared with insertion of an oesophageal stent in the palliative setting. Brachytherapy is usually performed without general anaesthetic and as a day case procedure, which makes it an appealing treatment option for patients. Guidelines for its use in oesophageal cancer have been produced by the American Brachytherapy Society (Gaspar et al., 1997). The treatment involves the use of a radioactive material, usually iridium-192, and is passed down the oesophagus to the level of the tumour.

13. A Achalasia

Gastric polyps are usually asymptomatic and found incidentally. Large polyps may present with bleeding, anaemia, abdominal discomfort or gastric outlet obstruction. A classification of polyps is given in **Table 7.1**.

Fundic gland polyps are usually multiple transparent sessile polyps, 1–5 mm in diameter, located in the body and fundus. They are not associated with atrophic gastritis and the prevalence of *Helicobacter pylori* infection is very low in these patients.

Gastric adenomas are true neoplasms and are precursors of gastric cancer. Histologically, they are classified as tubular, villous and tubulovillous types. They are often solitary and can be found anywhere in the stomach but are commonly found in the antrum. They frequently arise on a background of atrophic gastritis and intestinal metaplasia, but there is no proven association with *H. pylori* infection.

Up to 80% of hyperplastic polyps have been found to regress after eradication of *H. pylori* before endoscopic removal.

Table 7.1 Classification of gastric polyps	
Epithelial polyps	**Nonmucosal intramural polyps**
Fundic gland polyp	Gastrointestinal stromal tumour
Hyperplastic polyp	Leiomyoma
Adenomatous polyp	Inflammatory fibroid polyp
Hamartomatous polyp:	Fibroma and fibromyoma
• Juvenile polyp	Lipoma
• Peutz–Jeghers syndrome	Ectopic pancreas
• Cowden's syndrome	Neurogenic and vascular tumours
Polyposis syndromes (nonhamartomatous):	Neuroendocrine tumours (carcinoids)
• Juvenile polyposis	
• Familial adenomatous polyposis	

14. C Forceful dilatation of the oesophagus with a balloon can produce excellent results

Achalasia can be treated with the injection of botulinum toxin into the lower oesophageal sphincter, which causes the sphincter to relax via the same mechanism by which it produces the cosmetic effects on facial muscles. Other possible treatment options include pneumatic dilatation which has also been shown to produce excellent results and can provide relief of symptoms in 70–90% of patients for more than 1 year. A Cochrane review has demonstrated that pneumatic dilatation has better outcomes than botulinum injections (Leyden et al., 2006).

15. B Pulsion diverticulae are most common in the distal oesophagus

Oesophageal diverticulae can be diagnosed within any part of the oesophagus, with the pulsion type being far more common than traction diverticulum. Pulsion diverticulae arise more commonly in the distal oesophagus, on the right posterolateral wall. These are also known as epiphrenic diverticulum. The most common symptoms which arise from oesophageal diverticulum are dysphagia, regurgitation and pneumonia which occurs from aspiration into the lungs. Barium swallow and/or upper gastrointestinal endoscopy are both useful to diagnose the diverticulum.

16. D Type IV

The woman has a type IV gastric ulcer (**Table 7.2**).

Table 7.2 Types of gastric ulcer	
Ulcer type	**Location**
Type I	Body of stomach, most often lesser curve
Type II	Body of stomach in combination with duodenal ulceration
Type III	Pyloric channel within 3 cm of the pylorus
Type IV	Gastroesophageal
Type V	Any location associated with NSAID use

17. B 5

The risk scoring system developed by Rockall et al. 1966 (see **Table 1.14**) is a clinical scoring system for managing patients with acute upper gastrointestinal bleeds. It categorises patients as low and high-risk for mortality if they have had such a bleed. This 55-year-old has a Rockall score of 5, which is calculated as follows:

Age – 0

Shock – 2 (systolic <100 mmHg)

Comorbidities – 0

Diagnosis – 1 (ulcer)

Major stigmata of recent haemorrhage – 2 (visible clot)

18. E Gastrectomy is always required

Ménétrier's disease presents with abdominal pain, nausea and vomiting and peripheral oedema secondary to protein losing gastropathy. It is characterised by large rugal folds of the fundus and body of the stomach. The antrum is usually spared. These can be seen on fluoroscopic or CT imaging, or at endoscopy. Full thickness biopsies are required for diagnosis. Histology shows foveolar hyperplasia, tortuous (corkscrew) and cystically dilated foveolar glands. Some cases show marked intraepithelial lymphocytosis and glandular atrophy, evident as hypoplasia of parietal and chief cells.

Cetuximab, a monoclonal antibody against epidermal growth factor receptor is first line treatment. Gastrectomy may be required for those who do not respond or continue to have severe protein loss.

19. B Boerhaave's syndrome

The classical triad is described as chest pain associated with vomiting and clinical examination may reveal subcutaneous emphysema. As in this 42-year-old patient, sufferers may be extremely unwell and in shock. Rapid resuscitation is required, with intensive therapy unit support and oral water-soluble contrast radiography is the gold standard investigation. Treatment depends on a number of factors but thoracotomy (usually on the left side due to this being the frequent side of perforation) and closure of the perforation or simple drainage are the main options.

20. E *Trypanosoma cruzi*

Chagas' syndrome is a tropical parasitic disease caused by the protozoa *Trypanosoma cruzi*. It is responsible for ongoing gastrointestinal symptoms because of its effects on the enteric nervous system. Chagas' syndrome can be acute or chronic, depending on the presence of the parasite. *Pseudomonas aeruginosa* is a bacterium that is found is the soil and causes opportunistic infections in humans – especially the immunocompromised.

Answer: EMIs

21. L Splenic hilum

Station 10 gastric lymph nodes represent the splenic hilum nodes.

22. G Lesser curvature nodes

Station 3 gastric lymph nodes represent the nodes along the lesser curvature of the stomach.

23. C Hepatoduodenal ligament nodes

Station 12 gastric lymph nodes represent the nodes along the hepatoduodenal ligament.

24. A Coeliac nodes

Station 9 gastric lymph nodes represent the coeliac artery nodes.

25. K Root of mesentery nodes

Station 14 gastric lymph nodes represent the nodes at the root of the mesentery.

26. E Left gastric artery nodes

Station 7 gastric lymph nodes represent the nodes along the left gastric artery.

27. C Boerhaave's syndrome

This is a common finding in Boerhaave's syndrome which normally presents as a sudden rupture of the oesophagus with associated perforation. Contamination through the perforation is usually into the left side of the thorax. If surgery is undertaken, the findings are usually a solitary tear in the oesophagus on the left, posterolateral position. It must also be remembered that it is important to extend the muscular incision at the time of repair as the inner mucosal injury is usually greater.

28. A Black oesophagus syndrome

Black oesophagus syndrome is an uncommon condition of which the cause has not yet been identified, but venous thrombosis is the most likely reason. As the name suggests it is identified by black discolouration of the entire oesophageal mucosa. Patients will be extremely unwell.

29. J Stent placement

Oesophageal stenting has the highest risk of iatrogenic perforation of the oesophagus with reported rates of 5–25%. Although oesophageal stents have been documented to offer acceptable palliation for patients with advanced oesophageal cancer, complications because of stent migration, occlusion of the stent and recurrent dysphagia are proven and therefore must be discussed with patients prior to them undergoing such interventions.

30. D First degree caustic burn

This is the description of endoscopy findings of first-degree oesophageal caustic injury. There is hyperaemia only with only mild mucosal oedema and no mucosal loss.

31. K Third degree caustic burn

This is the description of the endoscopic findings for third degree oesophageal caustic injury. There is moderate to severe bleeding and severe oedema with deep ulcers. Eschar is only present though in late endoscopy findings.

32. I Second degree caustic burn

This situation describes the endoscopic findings in second degree oesophageal caustic injury with mild to moderate bleeding, moderate oedema and mucosal ulceration or blistering.

33. L Systemic sclerosis

This 34-year-old man has the characteristic cutaneous appearances of skin thickening and oedema in affected individuals with systemic sclerosis. Up to 80% of affected patients will also have signs of the disease in their oesophagus, which leads to smooth muscle atrophy involving the lower oesophageal sphincter.

34. E Nutcracker oesophagus

These are the findings on oesophageal manometry (with high amplitude oesophageal contractions) that are associated with nutcracker oesophagus, which this patient has a diagnosis of.

35. K Secondary achalasia

Chronic infection with the parasite *Trypanosoma cruzi* causes Chagas' disease. This leads to similar symptoms seen in primary achalasia, but is itself a cause of secondary achalasia. Outside South America, the most common reason for secondary achalasia is a tight gastro-oesophageal junction following antireflux surgery.

36. G Primary achalasia

This is the classic histological finding of primary achalasia. It is due to progressive loss of ganglion cells in the myenteric plexus.

37. C Diverticulum

Oesophageal diverticulum can be found at any site in the oesophagus with the pulsion type being far more common than traction diverticulum. Pulsion diverticulae arise more frequently in the distal oesophagus occurring on the posterolateral wall of the oesophagus, with a tendency to be found on the right side.

38. B Diffuse oesophageal spasm

This 69-year-old woman demonstrates the classical features of diffuse oesophageal spasm on manometry studies. Diffuse oesophageal spasm has an unknown aetiology and patients typically present with chest pain and dysphagia. Findings on manometry include uncoordinated contractions in the smooth muscle layers of the oesophagus.

39. J Total gastrectomy

This patient requires a total gastrectomy. He has been found to have a proximal third gastric cancer and the current evidence from a Western population suggests that a total gastrectomy should be performed.

40. I Subtotal gastrectomy

The current standard of care for gastric cancers arising in the lower half of the stomach is to perform a subtotal gastrectomy. Currently in the Western world, evidence for more radical total gastrectomy is limited and the standard of treatment is a subtotal gastrectomy. This obviously has lower morbidity and mortality than total gastrectomy.

41. K Total gastrectomy with en-bloc distal pancreaticosplenectomy

This patient requires total gastrectomy and splenectomy. She is a 55-year-old woman who is fit and well, having been found to have locally advanced gastric cancer with direct of the tail of the pancreas. Staging reveals no distant disease in the liver or the lungs. Her only option for a curative resection is total gastrectomy and en-bloc distal pancreaticosplenectomy.

42. H Stenting

This 67-year-old patient requires palliation of his obstructing metastatic oesophageal cancer. Insertion of an oesophageal stent is a considered option but possible complications such as perforation and stent migration must be discussed with the patient preprocedure. A randomised study has shown that a single dose of brachytherapy may give better long-term palliation than insertion of a metal stent and this should also be considered (Sur et al. 1998).

43. D Gastrojejunostomy

This 78-year-old patient will have gastric outlet obstruction from his advanced distal gastric cancer which has been deemed inoperable. Formation of a gastrojejunostomy is required to allow palliation of his symptoms of vomiting.

44. G Radiotherapy

Definitive radiotherapy should be offered to this unfit woman, for relief of the symptoms caused by proximal oesophageal cancer. She is 75 years old and has been declared not fit for an anaesthetic, so radiotherapy treatment in this setting would be the most appropriate treatment. It may even offer an excellent outcome, especially in view of the fact this is a proximal cancer which will be squamous cell and therefore radiosensitive.

45. C Cisplatin only

Cisplatin causes renal toxicity. It has multiple cellular effects which lead to tubular damage and loss of sodium, potassium and magnesium. In some patients this damage will cause an irreversible reduction in glomerular filtration rate but in others the effect is reversible.

46. L Taxane only

These are both taxanes. Taxanes are extremely toxic drugs sometimes reserved for the treatment of advanced upper gastrointestinal cancers in the form of second line treatment. Side effects include bone marrow suppression and peripheral neuropathy. The COUGAR-02 trial (Ford et al, 2014), a randomised controlled trial comparing docetaxel or active symptom control (radiotherapy, steroids, supportive medications) deemed necessary by the treating physician in patients with locally advanced or metastatic oesophagogastric adenocarcinoma who had progressed despite previous platinum–fluropyrimidine chemotherapy, showed an improved overall survival in the docetaxel group.

47. A Brachytherapy

Studies have suggested that brachytherapy is a good treatment for the palliation of symptoms in oesophageal cancer. Brachytherapy is usually performed without general anaesthetic and as a day case procedure. Guidelines for its use in oesophageal cancer have been produced by the American Brachytherapy Society (Gaspar et al., 1997). The process involves the use of a radioactive material, usually iridium-192, which is passed down the oesophagus to the level of the tumour.

48. E Epirubicin, cisplatin and continuous-infusion 5-fluorouracil (ECF) regimen

The UK Medical Research Council MAGIC trial (Cunningham et al, 2006) compared surgery alone with perioperative ECF and surgery in patients with potentially resectable gastric, oesophagogastric or distal oesophageal adenocarcinomas. In those undergoing perioperative ECF, tumours were of decreased size and stage, and progression-free, and overall survival was improved.

49. B Capecitabine, cisplatin and trastuzumab

The ToGA trial (Bang et al, 2010) compared chemotherapy alone and chemotherapy with trastuzumab in the treatment of patients with advanced gastric or oesophagogastric tumours showing HER-2 protein overexpression. The group receiving trastuzumab has increased overall survival.

50. K External bean radiotherapy, paclitaxel and carboplatin

The CROSS trial (van Hagen et al, 2012) compared preoperative chemoradiotherapy with surgery alone in patients with potentially resectable oesophageal or oesophagogastric tumours. Survival was significantly improved in those receiving pre-operative chemoradiotherapy.

Chapter 8

Vascular and endovascular surgery

Questions: SBAs

For each question, select the single best answer from the five options listed.

1. A 44-year-old woman is diagnosed with left-sided thoracic outlet symptoms.

   What are the symptoms of thoracic outlet syndrome (TOS) most commonly due to?

   A Arterial TOS
   B Neurogenic TOS
   C Non-specific (combined) TOS
   D Positional TOS
   E Venous TOS

2. A 59-year-old man with insulin-dependent diabetes presents with a hot erythematous swollen right foot. There is no history of pain or any injury. There is a palpable posterior tibial pulse but no dorsalis pedis pulse and there are no obvious breaks in the skin. Plain radiography suggests some fragmented subchondral bone in the midfoot. Inflammatory markers are within normal limits.

   What is the most likely diagnosis?

   A Charcot's foot
   B Critical limb ischaemia
   C Deep venous thrombosis
   D Osteomyelitis
   E Superficial cellulitis

3. A 66-year-old man has undergone a left carotid endarterectomy and develops symptoms as a result of an iatrogenic nerve injury. Damage to which of the following nerves would result in the accompanying neurological deficit?

   A Facial nerve, resulting in drooping of the contralateral corner of the mouth
   B Glossopharyngeal nerve, resulting in difficulty in swallowing
   C Hypoglossal nerve, resulting in altered taste
   D Superior laryngeal nerve, resulting in hoarseness and loss of effective cough
   E Vagus nerve, resulting in diaphragmatic paralysis

4. A 34-year-old man is diagnosed with Buerger's disease (thromboangiitis obliterans).

    What is the diagnosis of Buerger's disease reliant upon?

    A   A positive serum antineutrophil cytoplasmic antibody
    B   Exclusion of other causes
    C   Large vessel angiographic changes
    D   Raised erythrocyte sedimentation rate
    E   Resolution of symptoms with antiplatelet therapy

5. A 22-year-old woman has marked lymphoedema in her right leg.

    What is the most appropriate management?

    A   Diuretic therapy
    B   Elevation and elastic support stockings
    C   Excision of scarred skin and fibrotic subcutaneous tissue
    D   Lymphatic bypass
    E   Massage therapy or mechanical compression

6. A 65-year-old woman has a graft infection following a femoropopliteal bypass
    (using a prosthetic graft).

    What is most likely causative organism?

    A   *Escherichia coli*
    B   *Haemophilus*
    C   *Pseudomonas*
    D   *Staphylococcus*
    E   *Streptococcus*

7. A 68-year-old woman with known peripheral vascular disease presents with a
    12-hour history of right foot and calf pain. Her pulseless foot has fixed mottling is
    and insensate from her ankle distally. She can move her ankle with some discomfort
    in her tender swollen calf, but she has no movement in her midfoot or toes.

    What is the Rutherford's classification (and prognosis)?

    A   Immediately threatened (Rutherford class IIa ischaemia)
    B   Irreversibly ischaemic (Rutherford class III ischaemia)
    C   Marginally threatened (Rutherford class I ischaemia)
    D   Marginally threatened (Rutherford class IIa ischaemia)
    E   Unsalvageable and an amputation is required (Rutherford class IV ischaemia)

8. A 27-year-old man has been found to have a left-sided carotid body tumour.

    Which of the following statements does not describe tumours of the carotid body?

    A   The tumours arise from paraganglion cells
    B   They are commonly benign
    C   They are commonly familial
    D   They are mobile side-to-side
    E   They are hard solid, painless highly vascular tumours

9. A 19-year-old woman undergoes an endoscopic thoracic sympathectomy at T2 and
   T3 levels for palmar hyperhidrosis.

   What is the most common significant side effect of this procedure?

   A   Cardiac sympathetic denervation
   B   Compensatory sweating
   C   Failure of the procedure (residual symptoms of hyperhidrosis)
   D   Gustatory sweating
   E   Horner's syndrome

10. A 55-year-old man undergoes an elective endovascular aneurysm repair. Within
    3 hours he becomes haemodynamically unstable and an urgent CT angiogram
    reveals a leak of contrast between the main body of the graft and the left limb
    extension.

    What is the most likely diagnosis?

    A   Type I endoleak
    B   Type II endoleak
    C   Type III endoleak
    D   Type IV endoleak
    E   Type V endoleak

11. A 67-year-old man has a right popliteal aneurysm diagnosed by his attending
    surgeon, following endovascular repair of a 7 cm abdominal aortic aneurysm.

    When would repair of the popliteal aneurysm not be indicated?

    A   A 1.7 cm popliteal aneurysm with distal embolisation
    B   A 1.8 cm popliteal aneurysm with new calf swelling
    C   A 1.9 cm popliteal aneurysm with right buttock pain
    D   A 3.1 cm popliteal aneurysm which is asymptomatic
    E   A 3.7 cm popliteal aneurysm with right calf claudication

12. A 68-year-old woman presents to the emergency department with a history of
    right-sided amaurosis fugax approximately 10 days ago. Subsequently, a carotid
    duplex shows 70% left internal carotid artery stenosis and 70% right internal artery
    stenosis. CT angiogram confirms this finding with both vertebral arteries being
    patent.

    Which of the following is the recommended management?

    A   Right carotid endarterectomy
    B   Left carotid endarterectomy
    C   75 mg clopidogrel and 80 mg atorvastatin
    D   Right carotid artery stenting
    E   Left carotid artery stenting

13. A 57-year-old man has lifestyle-limiting subclavian steal syndrome.

Which of the following is not an appropriate treatment option?

A   Carotid-subclavian bypass
B   Medical management
C   Percutaneous transluminal angioplasty
D   Subclavian-carotid transposition
E   Subclavian endarterectomy

14. A 63-year-old woman develops a left-sided deep vein thrombosis and is felt to have a hypercoagulable state.

Which of the following is not associated with hypercoagulability?

A   Antiphospholipid syndrome
B   Antithrombin III deficiency
C   Factor V Leiden deficiency
D   Heparin-induced thrombocytopaenia
E   Protein S deficiency

15. A 52-year-old man in the coronary care unit requires emergency thrombolysis.

Which of the following is an absolute contraindication to thrombolysis?

A   Coarctation of the aorta
B   Hypertension (165/90 mmHg)
C   LeFort III fracture 9 months ago
D   Previous gastrectomy for bleeding gastric ulcer 8 months ago
E   Previous intracranial bleed 12 months ago

16. A 77-year-old woman undergoes a CT of the abdomen to stage her colorectal cancer. This identifies an incidental visceral artery aneurysm.

Which artery does a visceral arterial aneurysm occur most commonly in?

A   Coeliac
B   Hepatic
C   Inferior mesenteric
D   Splenic
E   Superior mesenteric

17. A 22-year-old man develops compartment syndrome in his left calf following a closed tibial fracture.

Which compartment is most commonly affected by compartment syndrome?

A   Anterior compartment
B   Deep posterior compartment
C   Lateral compartment
D   Peroneal compartment
E   Superficial posterior compartment

18. A 79-year-old man presents with a thoracoabdominal aortic aneurysm (TAA) originating at the level of his diaphragm and extending to the aortic bifurcation.

What classification of TAA is this?

A   Crawford III
B   Crawford IV
C   DeBakey type II
D   DeBakey type III
E   Stanford type B

19. Following endothelial injury several growth factors and adhesion molecules are implicated in the restenotic process.

Which of the following markers is not associated with the process of restenosis?

A   E-selectin
B   Intracellular adhesion molecule-1
C   Platelet derived growth factor
D   Vascular endothelial growth factor
E   von Willebrand factor

20. A 59-year-old woman has pain after eating which is attributed to mesenteric ischaemia.

Which of the following conditions is not a recognised cause of mesenteric ischaemia?

A   Atherosclerosis
B   Median arcuate ligament syndrome
C   Nutcracker syndrome (mesoaortic compression)
D   Takayasu's arteritis
E   Thromboangiitis obliterans

21. A 62-year-old man has had an ischaemic stroke 5 days previously. A duplex scan reveals a symptomatic 80% stenosis and he is now classified as a Rankin grade 1.

Which of the following is not a recommended treatment option?

A   Carotid endarterectomy within 48 hours
B   Carotid endarterectomy within 2 weeks
C   Commence aspirin 300 mg
D   Commence aspirin and clopidogrel
E   Commence high-dose statin

Questions: EMIs

Theme: Vascular treatment modalities

A   Aortobifemoral bypass
B   Axillobifemoral bypass
C   Exercise therapy
D   Femoral embolectomy
E   Femorodistal bypass
F   Femorofemoral crossover
G   Femoropopliteal bypass

H   Forefoot amputation
I   Iliac stenting
J   Intravenous heparin
K   Syme's amputation
L   Transfemoral amputation
M   Transtibial amputation

Instructions: For each of the following scenarios, choose the single most appropriate treatment from the list above. Each option may be used once, more than once or not at all.

22. A 68-year-old man presents with dry gangrene of the left hallux. He takes clopidogrel and atorvastatin, started by his GP. He is a heavy smoker. At night he tells you the foot keeps him awake and for the last 3 weeks, he has been sleeping in a chair. On examination, he has a good femoral pulse but nothing palpable distally. MR angiogram shows a full length superficial femoral artery occlusion. The popliteal artery is patent below the knee and there is single-vessel anterior tibial runoff distally.

23. A 52-year-old woman presents with a 3-month history of a numb right foot. Prior to that she could only walk 50 m before having to stop due to pain in the right calf. On examination, she has no pulses palpable in the right leg. The left leg has a full complement of pulses palpable. Angiogram reveals a 2-cm occlusion of the mid right common iliac artery. The left iliac system is patent.

24. An 89-year-old woman presents with gangrene of the tips of the toes of both feet. She has previously had an aortobifemoral bypass carried out 15 years ago. She lives independently but is frail. On examination, she has no pulses palpable in either lower limb. CT angiogram reveals aortic occlusion at the level of the renal arteries. The aortobifemoral bypass is occluded. The common femoral arteries, profunda femoris arteries and superficial femoral arteries are patent. The popliteal arteries also appear patent with 3-vessel runoff bilaterally.

Theme: CEAP classification of venous incompetence

A   C0 Ep
B   C1 Ep
C   C1 Es
D   C2 Ep
E   C2 Es
F   C3 Ep
G   C3 Es

H   C4 Ep
I   C4 Es
J   C5 Ep
K   C5 Es
L   C6 Ep
M   C6 Es

Instructions: For each of the following scenarios, choose the single most likely CEAP classification from the list above. Each option may be used once, more than once or not at all.

25. A 75-year-old woman has had varicose veins for 50 years. She has developed an ulcer over her medial gaiter area. Duplex scanning shows mild stenosis of the superficial femoral artery in the adductor canal. Ankle brachial pressure index is 0.85. Venous duplex shows reflux in the great saphenous vein, the deep system is competent.

26. A 25-year-old man has right sided varicose veins in the distribution of the short saphenous vein. He has no skin changes. The varicosities have been present for the last 4 years. Venous duplex shows reflux in the short saphenous vein. The great saphenous vein and deep venous system are patent and competent.

27. A 59-year-old woman has lipodermatosclerosis of the left gaiter region. Venous duplex shows reflux in the great saphenous vein. She has previously had a left ankle fracture which required internal fixation 15 years ago. Postoperatively, she was treated for thrombosis of the superficial femoral vein.

Theme: Serious side effects

A   Acute renal failure
B   Addison's disease
C   Acute respiratory distress syndrome
D   Cardiomyopathy
E   Cholelithiasis
F   Intracranial haemorrhage
G   Lactic acidosis

H   Myopathy
I   Nephrogenic systemic fibrosis
J   Peptic ulcer disease
K   Retroperitoneal fibrosis
L   Rhabdomyolysis
M   Thrombocytopaenia

Instructions: For each of the following drugs, choose the single most likely side effect from the list above. Each option may be used once, more than once or not at all.

28. Heparin.

29. Simvastatin.

30. Gadolinium.

Theme: Eponymous conditions

A Behçet's disease
B Charcot's disease
C Churg–Strauss syndrome
D Ehlers–Danlos syndrome
E Loeys–Dietz syndrome
F Marfan's syndrome
G Milroy's disease
H Osler–Weber–Rendu syndrome
I Paget–Schroetter syndrome
J Parkes–Weber syndrome
K Sturge–Weber syndrome
L Takayasu's disease
M Wegener's granulomatosis

Instructions: For each of the following scenarios, choose the single most likely diagnosis from the list above. Each option may be used once, more than once or not at all.

31. A 12-year-old girl presents with bilateral lower limb swelling. There is pitting oedema to the knee bilaterally. There is no history of trauma and the parents describe her legs as being 'quite puffy' for the last few years.

32. A 45-year-old man is referred to the vascular clinic with superficial thrombophlebitis after a diagnosis of systemic vasculitis is made in the community. There is a past medical history which includes aphthous ulcers, genital ulcers, and uveitis.

33. A 29-year-old man has a new swelling of the left arm extending from his hand to his axilla. This occurred after he had been lifting weights in the gym.

Theme: Renal access

A Brachioaxillary polytetrafluoroethylene (PTFE) graft
B Brachiocephalic fistula
C Distal revascularisation-interval ligation (DRIL)
D Femoral line insertion
E Gracz fistula
F Necklace graft
G Peritoneal dialysis
H Radial basilic fistula
I Snuffbox fistula
J Thigh loop graft
K Transposed branchiobasilic fistula
L Tunnelled central venous catheter
M Ulnocephalic fistula

Instructions: For each of the following scenarios, choose the single most likely access from the list above. Each option may be used once, more than once or not at all.

34. A 68-year-old woman (who is right-hand dominant) has had previous left radiocephalic and brachiocephalic fistulae which have both failed because of multiple stenotic lesions in her left cephalic vein. Duplex scanning reveals no other arterial or venous pathology in any of her four limbs.

35. A 70-year-old man with type 1 diabetes has newly diagnosed aortoiliac disease and is noted to have a gangrenous right 5th finger and gangrenous tips to his left 4th and 5th fingers. Despite this he has never been in hospital before, but his GP has recently noted abnormally high urea and creatinine on routine biochemistry. His renal function is progressively worsening and he is expected to require dialysis in the next few weeks.

36. A 44-year-old man with multiple previous abdominal operations is predialysis but is keen to avoid prolonged periods in hospital. The renal physicians are looking for an access option prior to dialysis in the next 2–3 months. He has excellent quality arteries and veins in both arms.

Theme: Investigations

A Ankle brachial pressure index
B Arterial duplex
C Carotid Doppler
D Cardiopulmonary exercise testing
E Chest X-ray
F CT of brain
G Computed tomography angiography

H Digital subtraction angiography
I Echocardiogram
J Multiple gated acquisition scan
K Magnetic resonance angiography
L Pulmonary function tests
M Venous duplex
N White cell scan

Instructions: For each of the following scenarios, choose the single most likely investigation from the list above. Each option may be used once, more than once or not at all.

37. A 70-year-old man has a 7 cm abdominal aortic aneurysm and the anaesthetist has concerns over his cardiovascular and respiratory systems. After routine tests are performed the anaesthetist requests a non-invasive assessment of the patient's functional exercise capacity.

38. An 89-year-old woman has long-standing venous eczema in her right gaiter area and has now developed an ulcer. There is no history of trauma, but she has bilateral ankle and feet swelling. Her medical history includes exertional angina and warfarinisation for atrial fibrillation.

39. A 62-year-old man who had a previous transient ischaemic attack 1 year ago is due to undergo coronary artery bypass grafting in the next 3 months.

Theme: Amputation types

A Burgess
B Chopart
C Digital
D Lisfranc
E Gritti–Stokes
F Hindquarter
G Ray

H Skew-flap
I Syme's
J Through knee
K Transfemoral
L Transmetatarsal
M Transtibial

Instructions: For each of the following scenarios, choose the single most appropriate amputation from the list above. Each option may be used once, more than once or not at all.

40. A 44-year-old man with insulin-dependent diabetes has spreading infection in his foot originating from a necrotic hallux. Plain radiographs demonstrate osteomyelitis of the first metatarsal head.

41. A 27-year-old woman required a through-ankle amputation following a road traffic accident. Her amputation has an excellent end-bearing stump on the distal tibia and fibula with a prominent fat pad.

42. A 49-year-old man with a history of intravenous drug abuse and type 2 diabetes underwent amputation of his right second toe but now has to undergo a further amputation because of spreading infection. On marking his leg the attending surgeon notices ascending lymphangitis.

Theme: Leg pain

A	Cystic adventitial disease	H	Phlegmasia cerulea dolens
B	Embolic	I	Popliteal entrapment syndrome
C	Klippel–Trenaunay syndrome	J	Rheumatoid arthritis
D	Leriche's syndrome	K	Sciatica
E	May–Thurner syndrome	L	Superficial femoral artery occlusion
F	Mixed connective tissue disease	M	Takayasu's arteritis
G	Osteoarthritis	N	Thromboangiitis obliterans

Instructions: For each of the following scenarios, choose the single most likely diagnosis from the list above. Each option may be used once, more than once or not at all.

43. A 25-year-old man describes pain in his right calf when exercising which resolves with cessation of activity. He has a full complement of pulses. He is investigated by the orthopaedic surgeons who arrange an MRI of his knee, which is subsequently reportedly as normal.

44. A 65-year-old woman presents with left thigh and calf pain and swelling. There is no obvious discolouration. A venogram suggests there is fresh thrombus in the left common iliac vein. The patient is otherwise well, with no history of trauma or immobility, recent travel or hormone replacement therapy.

45. A 58-year-old man complains of buttock claudication and progressive impotence. His claudication slightly improves following smoking cessation and commencing aspirin and statin therapy.

Theme: Arterial pathologies

A	Adrenal artery	H	Middle cerebral artery
B	Anterior cerebral artery	I	Ophthalmic artery
C	Coeliac artery	J	Posterior cerebral artery
D	Common iliac artery	K	Renal arcuate artery
E	Gastroduodenal artery	L	Superficial temporal artery
F	Inferior mesenteric artery	M	Superior mesenteric artery
G	Internal iliac artery		

Instructions: For each of the following scenarios, choose the single most likely involved artery from the list above. Each option may be used once, more than once or not at all.

46. A 45-year-old woman has median arcuate ligament syndrome.

47. A 66-year-old man develops a type II endoleak following an elective standard endovascular aneurysm repair.

48. An 88-year-old man has a short history of amaurosis fugax.

Answers: SBAs

1. B Neurogenic TOS

Neurogenic thoracic outlet syndrome (TOS) is the most common form of TOS. Approximately 80–90% of TOS presents with neurogenic symptoms in the ulnar nerve root distribution. There is often no obvious anatomical abnormality present, although a cervical rib, muscular hypertrophy or fibrous band may be present. When a cervical rib is present (**Figure 8.1**) there is a visible reduction in the space between the first rib, clavicle and anterior and middle scalene muscles. This can cause pressure effects on the artery or nerves resulting in arterial or neurogenic TOS respectively. In the thoracic outlet, venous compression (Paget–Schroetter syndrome) is due to narrowing in the space between the first rib, clavicle and medial border of the anterior scalene muscle.

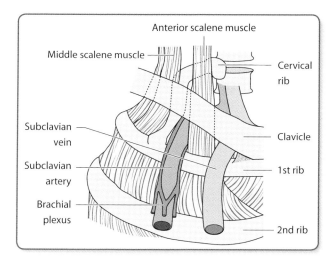

Figure 8.1 The thoracic outlet.

2. A Charcot's foot

Charcot's foot is a neuropathic arthropathy with degeneration of a weight-bearing joint (commonly tarsometatarsal or metatarsophalangeal joints). It usually has an insidious onset and manifests with bony destruction and resorption, and resulting deformity in the foot. Particular care must be taken when assessing diabetic foot problems as diabetic patients are 8–24 times more likely to have a major amputation than non-diabetics.

The clinical features of Charcot's foot may be mistaken for a sprain, gout, deep vein thrombosis, osteomyelitis or cellulitis. However, in any diabetic, neuropathic patient presenting with a red, hot, swollen foot with palpable pulses, Charcot's arthropathy should be the likeliest differential diagnosis, particularly in the absence of a soft tissue injury or portal of entry for infection. Local policy holders must decide between the two main investigative tools available (after plain radiographic imaging), MRI and FDG-PET, to help differentiate a Charcot's foot from osteomyelitis.

3. B Glossopharyngeal nerve, resulting in difficulty in swallowing

Each of the five nerves listed can be injured during carotid endarterectomy. However damage to cranial nerve (CN) VII, the facial nerve, would result in drooping of the ipsilateral corner of the mouth, if the marginal mandibular branch was affected. Injury to CNIX (the glossopharyngeal nerve) could result in difficulty in swallowing. A palsy of CNXII (the hypoglossal nerve) may result in deviation of the tongue to the ipsilateral side but would not affect taste which is supplied by the chordae tympani. Superior laryngeal nerve damage may affect voice quality and in particular may cause loss of high pitch phonation. At this level damage to CNX (the vagus nerve) could cause hoarseness or impaired cough and would not affect fibres to the diaphragm.

4. B Exclusion of other causes

The diagnosis of thromboangiitis obliterans is difficult as it is dependent upon on the exclusion of other conditions. Olin (2000) has proposed the following diagnostic criteria:

- Men between 20 and 40 years old
- History of tobacco use
- Distal extremity ischaemia (either claudication, rest pain ulcers or gangrene)
- Exclusion of other conditions including hypercoagulable states and diabetes mellitus
- Exclusion of a proximal source of emboli (by echocardiography and arterial imaging)
- Consistent arterial findings (including 'corkscrew' arteries) both in clinically involved and unaffected limbs

5. B Elevation and elastic support stockings

The vast majority of patients with lymphoedema have mild disease which can be successfully managed with leg elevation and elastic support stockings alone. Some patients will have moderate disease and may require mechanical pneumatic compression or massage therapy. Only a very small percentage of patients will progress to severe disease and may develop elephantiasis. In this group, operative intervention in the form of debulking surgery or lymphatic bypass may be considered.

6. D *Staphylococcus*

The rate of prosthetic graft infection ranges from 1–6% and debate continues over the correct course of management. There are exponents of both graft excision and graft salvage with long-term antibiotics. The Samson group have classified prosthetic graft infections on a scale from 1–5 (Samson et al., 1998), shown in **Table 8.1**.

The severity of the infection and the bacteriology available must be considered when deciding if graft salvage is possible. In a retrospective study of 42 major prosthetic graft infections (Samson group 3–5) observed over a 5-year period, Samson et al. (1998) cultured *Staphylococcus* in 50% of patients [n = 21; 10 *S. epidermidis*, 11 Methicillin-resistant *Staphylococcus aureus* (MRSA)]. The majority of the remainder were Gram- negative organisms (14; 3 *Pseudomonas*, 3 *Proteus* species, 2 *Escherichia coli* and 3 other). However, in 7 patients no organism was cultured. In this study, MRSA graft infection was associated with a significantly lower rate of graft salvage and limb salvage.

Table 8.1 Samson classification of prosthetic graft infection	
Group	**Definition of infection**
1	Confined to dermis
2	Involves subcutaneous tissue but does not make contact with graft
3	Involves body of graft but not anastomosis
4	Involves an exposed anastomosis but no bacteraemia/haemorrhage
5	Involves an exposed anastomosis plus bacteraemia and/or haemorrhage

7. B Irreversibly ischaemic (Rutherford class III ischaemia)

Clearly this patient has significant ischaemia and the reversibility of this will be determined by (i) the duration of her symptoms and (ii) her collateral blood supply. These factors will help determine how severe the tissue damage will be. If the mottling is fixed then the ischaemia is irreversible but from the above description it is unclear if this is the case. Profound paralysis and sensory loss is diagnostic of a non-viable limb but these can be subjective and open to varying interpretation. However, by the time the calf muscle becomes tender there is definitive dead muscle and the limb is therefore non-viable (**Table 8.2**). Options B and E both describe the correct prognosis but there is no class IV in Rutherford's classification system.

8. C They are commonly familial

Carotid body tumours (chemodectomas or carotid body paragangliomas) are highly vascular tumours arising from the paraganglion cells in the carotid body. They are located at the carotid bifurcation and characteristically splay the internal carotid

Table 8.2 Rutherford's classification of limb ischaemia						
Category	Description	Capillary return	Muscle paralysis	Sensory loss	Arterial Doppler	Venous Doppler
I Viable	Not immediately threatened	Intact	None	None	Audible	Audible
IIa Threatened (marginally)	Salvageable if treated promptly	Intact/ slow	None	Partial	Inaudible	Audible
IIb Threatened (immediately)	Salvageable if treated immediately	Slow/ absent	Partial, may have tender calf	Partial/ complete	Inaudible	Audible
III Irreversible	Unsalvageable	Absent	Complete, tense compartment	Complete	Inaudible	Inaudible

artery and external carotid artery. Like most paraganglionomas they are more common in women and are usually diagnosed in the fourth and fifth decades. Only a small proportion are familial (approximately 10%) and in such cases they are usually autosomal dominant in inheritance, and may be associated with neuroendocrine conditions such as MEN-2A and -2B, or von Hippel–Lindau.

Patients usually present with a slow growing spherical neck mass which may cause nerve palsies (involving vagus, glossopharyngeal or hypoglossal nerves). On examination the tumour may be moved side-to-side but not up or down, because of its fixed position within the carotid sheath. Like most paraganglionomas these tumours are normally benign (approximately 95%). Malignant transformation is uncommon (encountered in 2–36% of cases) and surgical excision is usually the treatment of choice. However, the larger the tumour, the greater the risk of operative complications and in patients for whom the risk of complications is too great, radiotherapy can be considered.

9. B Compensatory sweating

Endoscopic thoracic sympathectomy (ETS), or thoracoscopic sympathectomy, usually involves cauterising the thoracic ganglion (T2, T3 +/–T4) of the paraspinal sympathetic chain. It is a technique used when hyperhidrosis is refractory to medical management with aluminium chloride antiperspirants, anticholinergic drugs and botulinum toxin injections.

Following ETS, satisfaction rates of 80% have been quoted and relief from symptoms ranges from 85–95% of patients. The most common side effect of ETS is compensatory sweating, which was seen in 86% of 125 ETS patients followed-up over 3.8 years by the Gossot group in Paris (Gossot et al., 2003). Other less common side effects include gustatory sweating (<25%), cardiac sympathetic denervation (<5%), and Horner's syndrome (1–2%).

10. C Type III endoleak

Routine ultrasound or CT scanning may demonstrate continued sac expansion following endovascular aneurysm repair. This occurs due to ongoing leaking of blood into the aneurysm sac. This is termed an 'endoleak' of which there are five types.

- A type I endoleak is a failure of the sealing zone between the stent graft and the arterial wall. This can occur proximally at the (normally infrarenal) aneurysm neck or distally in either of the iliac limbs.
- A type II endoleak occurs when there is filling of the aneurysmal sac from patent side branches such as the lumbar arteries or inferior mesenteric artery.
- A type III endoleak is due to dislocation or separation of graft components.
- A type IV endoleak is due to graft porosity, and this is more evident around the time of the procedure when the patient is anticoagulated. This is a generally inconsequential and self-resolving phenomenon.
- A type V endoleak is also known as 'endotension', whereby arterial pulse pressure is transmitted into the arterial sac without any actual leak of the patient's blood. This is a contentious issue and many believe that endotension actually represents another form of endoleak which has previously been missed.

11. C A 1.9 cm popliteal aneurysm with right buttock pain

Popliteal aneurysms are present in 2–10% of patients with an abdominal aortic aneurysm (AAA). Additionally, in those who have a primary diagnosis of a popliteal aneurysm approximately 40% will have a coexisting AAA and 50% will have bilateral disease. Symptomatic popliteal aneurysms always require treatment and the most common symptomatic presentation is with distal embolisation or occlusion. Claudication and venous compression may also be presenting features. There are no firm guidelines for the management of asymptomatic popliteal aneurysms. However, many surgeons recommend intervention for aneurysms over 2 cm in size and most agree that it is mandatory for those over 3 cm. A 1.9 cm aneurysm is not sufficient in size to justify repair in the absence of any associated symptoms.

12. A Right carotid endarterectomy

This patient has symptomatic right carotid artery disease as shown on duplex and CT imaging. She requires secondary prevention as for all patients with arterial disease (antiplatelet, statin, blood pressure control, assessment for and management of diabetes and smoking cessation). She is within the timeframe (14 days) to achieve maximum benefit from carotid endarterectomy on the symptomatic diseased side (the right in this case) as she has 70% stenosis. Maximum benefit from carotid endarterectomy is seen in symptomatic patients with 70–99% stenosis within 2 weeks of symptom onset, but there is still a smaller benefit for symptomatic patients with >50% stenosis up to 6 weeks from onset of symptoms. Beyond this time point best medical management is recommended.

13. E Subclavian endarterectomy

Proximal subclavian lesions, either occlusions (**Figure 8.2**, A) or stenoses (**Figure 8.2**, B), can result in a decreased blood supply down the arm. During arm exercise this may cause blood to be diverted in a retrograde fashion down the vertebral artery beyond the occlusion or stenosis. This is known as 'subclavian steal' as blood from the circle of Willis is diverted to the subclavian artery. Most patients with such lesions are asymptomatic and therefore surgical treatment is not required. These patients can be successfully managed with control of modifiable risk factors and antiplatelet and statin therapy.

If patients develop symptoms due to subclavian steal, such as dizziness when exercising the ipsilateral limb, then interventional procedures may be merited. Angioplasty of the diseased segment is often the first line procedure, as it does not preclude subsequent surgical intervention and is less invasive. Both carotid-subclavian bypass and subclavian-carotid transposition procedures achieve resolution of symptoms in the majority of patients. Subclavian endarterectomy is not performed.

Figure 8.2 Subclavian lesions.

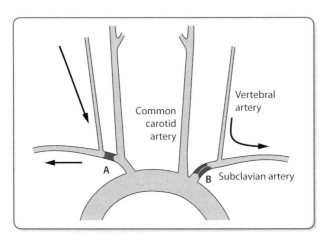

Common carotid artery

Vertebral artery

A

B   Subclavian artery

14. C Factor V Leiden deficiency

The coagulation cascade is composed of both intrinsic and extrinsic pathways. Factor V is activated by thrombin and acts as a cofactor with activated factor X to convert prothrombin to thrombin (**Figure 8.3**). Protein C and protein S both degrade factor V and consequently a deficiency of either protein C or S will result in a hypercoagulable state. Antiphospholipid syndrome inhibits protein C. Factor V Leiden is a mutated variant of factor V, which is not inactivated by protein C, and therefore results in a hypercoagulable state. It is the most common hereditary hypercoagulability disorder. Factor V Leiden deficiency is a misnomer.

Deficiency of Factor V exists, but this condition would result in decreased thrombin formation. Antithrombin III inactivates thrombin and a deficiency will lead to

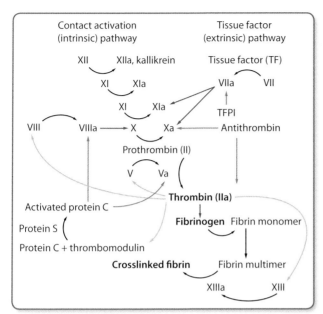

Figure 8.3 The coagulation cascade.

Within the figure:

Contact activation (intrinsic) pathway

Tissue factor (extrinsic) pathway

XII → XIIa, kallikrein

Tissue factor (TF)

XI → XIa

VIIa ← VII

XI → XIa

TFPI

VIII → VIIIa → X → Xa ← Antithrombin

Prothrombin (II)

V → Va

Thrombin (IIa)

Activated protein C

Fibrinogen → Fibrin monomer

Protein S

Protein C + thrombomodulin

Crosslinked fibrin ← Fibrin multimer

XIIIa ← XIII

hypercoagulability. Heparin-induced thrombocytopaenia (HIT) causes thrombosis despite a low platelet count. HIT predisposes to thrombosis despite a reduction in the platelet count.

15. E Previous intracranial bleed 12 months ago

Absolute contraindications to thrombolytic therapy include:

- Active bleeding (excluding menorrhagia)
- Aortic dissection
- Cerebral aneurysm or arteriovenous malformation
- Intracranial neoplasm
- Previous cerebral/intracranial haemorrhage (at any time)
- Recent thromboembolic stroke (within 3 months)

Relative contraindications include:

- Active peptic ulcer disease
- Bleeding diathesis (or current anticoagulant therapy)
- Pregnancy
- Recent head trauma (within 2–4 weeks)
- Recent gastrointestinal bleeding (within 6 months)
- Recent major surgery (within 2–3 weeks)
- Severe hypertension (>180/110 mmHg)

16. D Splenic

Visceral arterial aneurysms (VAA) were previously a very rare phenomenon but thanks to routine usage of high resolution imaging techniques (CT, MRI), they are now more frequently diagnosed. The commonest form of VAA is in the splenic artery, which accounts for 60–80% of cases. The hepatic artery is responsible for 20%, the superior mesenteric artery 6%, gastroduodenal and pancreatic 6%, coeliac 4%, gastric and gastroepiploic 4%, jejunal and ileocolic 3% and the inferior mesenteric artery occurs in <1%.

17. A Anterior compartment

There are three fascial compartments in the thigh (anterior, medial and posterior, **Figure 8.4**) and in the lower leg there are four (anterior, lateral, deep posterior and superficial posterior, **Figure 8.5**). The lateral compartment is also known as the peroneal compartment.

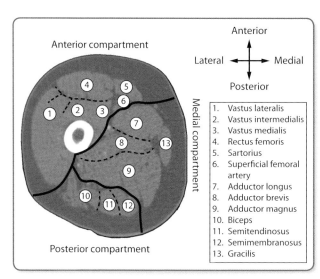

Figure 8.4 Compartments of the thigh.

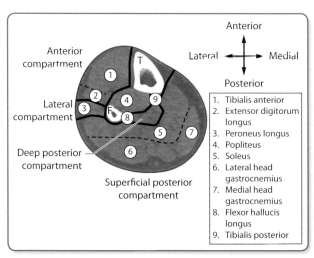

Figure 8.5 Compartments of the calf. T, tibia; F, fibia.

The anterior compartment is most commonly adversely affected by an increase in compartmental pressure both above and below the knee. The development of compartment syndrome is a clinical emergency and almost always mandates surgical fasciotomies. When compartment syndrome occurs there are symptoms of acute ischaemia with pain which is disproportionate, pallor, pulselessness, paraesthesia and even paralysis.

18. B Crawford IV

The Crawford classification is used to describe thoracoabdominal aortic aneurysms. It ranges from types I–IV (**Figure 8.6**).

> I – extends from the left subclavian artery to the suprarenal aorta
>
> II – extends from the left subclavian artery to the aortic bifurcation
>
> III – extends from the 6th rib/intercostal space to the aortic bifurcation
>
> IV – extends from the diaphragm to the aortic bifurcation
>
> V – extends from the 6th rib/intercostal space to the suprarenal aorta

The DeBakey and Stanford classifications are both used to describe aortic dissections (**Figure 8.7**). Stanford type A dissections originate in the ascending aorta (but can extend into the descending aorta) whereas type B only affect the descending aorta and originate distal to the left subclavian artery. The DeBakey classification further subclassifies Stanford A dissections into type 1 (involving the ascending and descending aorta in 10% of cases) and type 2 which is the most common (affecting the ascending aorta only in 60% of cases). Similar to Stanford type B, a DeBakey type 3 dissection involves the descending aorta only and occurs in the remaining 30%.

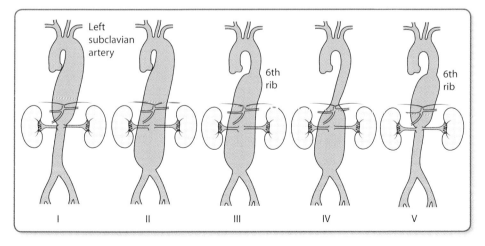

Figure 8.6 Crawford classification of thoracoabdominal aortic aneurysm.

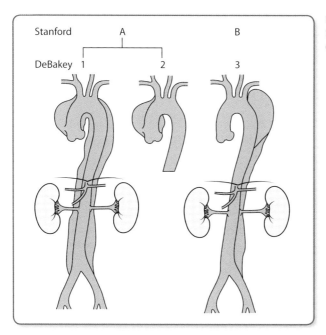

Figure 8.7 The DeBakey and Stanford classifications of aortic dissection.

19. D Vascular endothelial growth factor

Platelet-derived growth factor (PDGF) stimulates smooth muscle cell migration to the intima, which may result in intimal thickening and the development of a restenotic lesion. E-selectin is a cellular adhesion molecule which is associated with endothelial dysfunction, leukocyte recruitment and the development of restenosis. Intracellular adhesion molecule-1 mediates the adhesion and transmigration of leukocytes to the vascular endothelial wall and is vital in the initiation and progression of atherosclerosis and restenosis. von Willebrand factor (vWF) mediates platelet adhesion and increased levels of circulating vWF are linked to restenosis.

VEGF is an angiogenic factor which creates new blood vessels: (i) during embryonic development, (ii) after injury, and (iii) as part of collateralisation. It has been implicated in the re-endothelialisation of the vascular wall following percutaneous transluminal angioplasty and is thought to have a protective role against subsequent restenosis, by expediting the endothelial recovery.

20. C Nutcracker syndrome (mesoaortic compression)

The intestine is supplied by three vessels (the coeliac, superior mesenteric and inferior mesenteric arteries). However, symptoms of mesenteric ischaemia tend not to be present until two or more vessels are affected. The commonest cause of mesenteric ischaemia is atherosclerosis, although acute ischaemia can result from arterial thrombosis, acute embolism, venous thrombosis or 'non-occlusive' ischaemia. It is most commonly the superior mesenteric artery which is involved and may present with acute abdominal pain, nausea, vomiting or hypotension.

Median arcuate ligament syndrome occurs when the ligament causes compression of the coeliac axis with resulting symptoms. Patients with Takayasu's arteritis commonly have obstructive lesions of their visceral arteries but such patients are rarely symptomatic. Thromboangiitis obliterans (Buerger's disease) rarely affects mesenteric vessels and most of the literature involves case reports only.

Nutcracker syndrome (mesoaortic compression) affects the left renal vein whereby it is compressed between the abdominal aorta and the superior mesenteric artery.

21. D Commence aspirin and clopidogrel

The modified Rankin scale (mRS) is a used to measure the degree of disability or dependence in the daily activities of those who have suffered a stroke. It is a clinical outcome measure commonly used in stroke clinical trials.

In this patient's case he has no significant disability and would benefit from appropriate risk stratification and a timely carotid endarterectomy. There is no role for combination antiplatelet therapy with clopidogrel and aspirin [based on the most recent Scottish Intercollegiate Guidelines (2010) guidelines].

Answer: EMIs

22. G Femoropopliteal bypass

This man has critical limb ischaemia with tissue loss. He is still smoking and should be strongly advised to stop; however, his foot is threatened and he requires revascularisation. A long occlusion such as this would be best served with a bypass which would be femoral to below knee popliteal.

23. I Iliac stenting

This patient requires revascularisation as she has critical limb ischaemia. Her risk factors should be stratified and optimised. This is a short occlusion of the iliac system which should respond well to endovascular stenting. If the occlusion was flush to the aortic bifurcation kissing stents (right and left) may be required to ensure that the nonindex side is not compromised during stenting.

24. B Axillobifemoral bypass

This woman is elderly and frail. 'Re-do' aortic surgery would not be appropriate and therefore an axillobifemoral bypass would be the appropriate procedure for revascularisation.

25. L C6 Ep

This patient has an active venous ulcer (C6) with primary venous incompetence (Ep), no deep venous pathology (As) and the pathophysiology is reflux (Pr).

The CEAP classification (**Table 8.3**) is used to stratify varicose veins by severity, aetiology, distribution and cause, and aids description and communication for clinicians, specialists and researchers.

Table 8.3 The CEAP classification of venous incompetence			
C	**Clinical severity**	**E**	**Aetiology**
C0	No venous disease	Ec	Congenital
C1	Superficial (reticular) veins	Ep	Primary
C2	Truncal varicose veins	Es	Secondary
C3	Oedema	En	No venous cause
C4	Skin changes		
C5	Healed venous ulcer		
C6	Active venous ulcer		
A	**Anatomical distribution**	**P**	**Pathophysiology**
As	Superficial	Pr	Reflux
Ad	Deep	Po	Obstruction
Ap	Perforator	Pr,o	Both
An	No venous location	Pn	No venous pathophysiology

26. D C2 Ep

This man has truncal varicose veins (C2) that are primary (Ep), superficial (As) and the pathophysiology is reflux (Pr).

27. I C4 Es

This patient has venous skin changes (C4) due to the varicosities in the great saphenous vein. Due to the previous deep vein thrombosis this is a secondary phenomenon (Es).

28. M Thrombocytopaenia

Although heparin is used for the prevention of thrombosis, patients can occasionally develop heparin-induced thrombocytopaenia (HIT), where the platelet count falls below the normal range. Despite thrombocytopaenia, most patients with HIT will not experience any symptoms. However, patients can develop antibodies which result in increased platelet activation and this can lead to thrombosis despite the low platelet count.

29. H Myopathy

Approximately 1.5–3% of statin users in randomised controlled trials were shown to develop myalgia (Sathasivam & Lecky, 2008). In addition to myalgia, statin-induced muscle damage includes myositis, rhabdomyolysis, and increased creatine kinase levels.

30. I Nephrogenic systemic fibrosis

Nephrogenic systemic fibrosis (NSF) is a serious condition where skin, joints and internal organs develop excessive fibrosis leading to pain, contractures and organ failure. Several studies have associated the development of NSF with exposure to gadolinium, particularly in patients with established renal failure. This contrast agent is used in magnetic resonance angiography to evaluate patients for transplant suitability, demonstration of anatomy or for identification of post-transplant complications. As a result of this association, contrast which contains gadolinium is contraindicated in patients with an estimated glomerular filtration rate (eGFR) of less than 60 mL/min.

31. G Milroy's disease

Milroy's disease describes congenital lymphoedema which is characterised by idiopathic, painless oedema with pitting and skin changes (including hyperkeratosis). It is an autosomal dominant condition which results in limb swelling and leaves patients prone to cellulitis and infective episodes.

32. A Behçet's disease

Behçet's disease is an immune-mediated systemic vasculitis with a classical triad of aphthous ulcers, genital ulcers, and uveitis. Limb symptoms tend to be limited to superficial thrombophlebitis and joint pains.

33. I Paget–Schroetter syndrome

Paget–Schroetter is the condition of upper arm swelling because of venous obstruction in the axillary or subclavian vein. This can occur in patients with thoracic outlet syndrome where the vein is compressed between the anterior scale muscle and the space between the clavicle and the first rib (primary costoclavicular compression). **Figure 8.1** depicts the thoracic outlet. It is also associated with body-building (subclavius hypertrophy) and those with upper arm exertion because of axillary vein microtrauma.

34. K Transposed brachiobasilic fistula

The principles of arteriovenous (AV) fistula formation are that the primary creation of access should be in the non-dominant arm and sited as distally as possible. A snuffbox fistula is the most distal site followed by a radiocephalic (Brescia–Cimino) fistula. When a fistula fails the next access is normally attempted in the ipsilateral arm and again as distally as possible. Mid-forearm fistulas are created, if possible, prior to forming a brachiocephalic fistula in the antecubital fossa. The basilic vein can be subsequently used but requires transposition, to make it superficial enough to facilitate needling. A prosthetic graft may be used at later date to form a brachioaxillary graft in the non-dominant arm, although these have lower patency than autologous AV fistulae.

If both arms have no access options left, thigh loop grafts between the femoral artery and vein could be formed in either leg. In the presence of peripheral arterial disease of the lower legs, this is not possible as 'fistula steal' could result in a deterioration in arterial blood supply and the development of critical limb ischaemia. When all AV access options are exhausted, the decision between the patient, renal physician and surgeons is whether to continue with tunnelled central venous line dialysis or attempting peritoneal dialysis.

Peritoneal dialysis allows patients to dialyse at home through a catheter placed in the peritoneal cavity, but this technique is limited by the development of peritonitis and is not an option if there are adhesions or multiple previous abdominal operations.

In this patient's case, she has probably exhausted the cephalic vein in her non-dominant hand. The next step would be a basilic vein fistula (requiring transposition).

35. G Peritoneal dialysis

This man has aortoiliac disease and also has critical limb ischaemia in both arms. This would tend to preclude against an arteriovenous fistula. He should proceed to peritoneal dialysis.

36. I Snuffbox fistula

This man should have an arteriovenous fistula sited in his non-dominant arm as distally as possible. Although he seeks to avoid inpatient haemodialysis, he cannot have home peritoneal dialysis because of his multiple previous abdominal operations and the fact that he probably has adhesions. Assuming adequate arteries and veins, the best option would be a snuffbox fistula.

37. D CPEX

Cardiopulmonary exercise testing (CPEX or CPET) is now the 'gold standard' test for evaluating cardiopulmonary function. It is a non-invasive objective method of assessing the exercise response of the both the pulmonary and cardiovascular systems simultaneously.

38. A ABPI

Ankle brachial pressure index measurement is required to assess whether this patient can tolerate compression bandaging, because this is probably the mainstay of her treatment. It will also determine whether further investigation or treatment is required to improve arterial circulation to the affected area. A venous duplex would identify reflux, obstruction or thrombosis but the patient is already warfarinised and would not require additional antithrombotic treatment.

39. C Carotid Doppler

Carotid artery lesions (both intra- and extracranial) are an independent risk factor for central nervous system complications following coronary artery bypass grafting, and should be screened for as part of a preoperative assessment.

40. G Ray

A Ray amputation is performed at the level of the distal metatarsal head and for first and fifth toes this involves a 'racquet-shaped' incision. The extension of the 'racquet handle' along the medial or lateral border of the foot allows access to the neck of the metatarsal for bone division. This technique is commonly used in diabetic foot sepsis when there is extensive bony destruction and/or drainage of pus is required.

41. I Syme's

Syme originally described a through-ankle amputation which provides a durable end-bearing stump. It is an amputation through the dome of the tibia and is reliant on a good posterior tibial artery as the blood supply to the flap. The flap is formed from the subcalcaneal (heel) fat pad which is attached to the distal surface of the tibia.

42. A Burgess

All patients should have a vascular assessment prior to undergoing a lower limb amputation. Preserving the knee joint should allow 80% of previously ambulant patients to walk with a prosthesis. A Burgess type amputation involves a proximal tibial and fibular bone division with a long posterior myocutaneous flap. This well vascularised pedicle compensates for the poorly vascularised anterior skin flap. Studies examining the technique of skew-flaps have demonstrated no benefit over the established Burgess technique.

A Chopart amputation involves a disarticulation at the midtarsal joint and Lisfranc is a midfoot amputation.

43. I Popliteal entrapment syndrome

In popliteal entrapment syndrome there is abnormal anatomy in the popliteal fossa which may result in pressure effects on the popliteal artery. Normally the popliteal artery passes between the medial and lateral heads of gastrocnemius as it exits the popliteal fossa and trifurcates.

The commonest anatomical variant (**Figure 8.8**) is an abnormal insertion of the medial head of gastrocnemius which diverts, and impinges upon, the popliteal artery. This phenomenon is most common among young athletes when muscular hypertrophy may exacerbate compression of the popliteal artery.

Cystic adventitial disease presents in a similar group of patients but an MRI is likely to demonstrate the presence of a cystic structure on the outside of the artery.

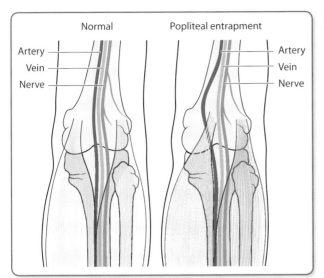

Figure 8.8 Popliteal entrapment syndrome.

44. E May–Thurner syndrome

May–Thurner syndrome occurs when the left common iliac vein is compressed by the overlying right common iliac artery. This syndrome can result in the development of a left ileofemoral deep vein thrombosis and should always be considered when there are no known prothrombotic factors. It is approximately three times more common in women and may require mechanical, as well as antithrombotic, therapy.

45. D Leriche's syndrome

Leriche's syndrome or aortoiliac disease presents as a classical triad of symptoms. It occurs most commonly in men with symptoms of buttock and thigh claudication, impotence and muscular atrophy.

46. C Coeliac artery

Compression of the coeliac artery (and coeliac ganglia) by the median arcuate ligament can result in mesenteric ischaemia and symptoms of abdominal pain. It is largely a diagnosis of exclusion and is further confounded by recurrence of symptoms following operative division of the ligament.

47. F Inferior mesenteric artery

A standard endovascular aneurysm repair encompasses the repair of an infrarenal abdominal aortic aneurysm. A type II endoleak involves continued bleeding into the aneurysm sac from a vessel between the sealing zones. This could either be due to a patent inferior mesenteric artery, or one of the lumbar arteries.

48.1 Ophthalmic artery

Amaurosis fugax is a transient monocular visual loss classically described as a 'curtain coming down in one eye'. When it is due to a vascular cause there is reduction in blood flow through the retinal or ophthalmic artery. The most common cause is embolic, from the ipsilateral internal carotid artery.

References

Abraczinskas DR, Ookubo R, Grace ND, et al. Propranolol for the prevention of first esophageal haemorrhage: a lifetime commitment? Hepatology 2001; 34:1096–1102.

Ain KB. Anaplastic thyroid carcinoma: a therapeutic challenge. Semin Surg Oncol 1999; 16:64–69.

American College of Chest Physicians (ACCP) and Society of Critical Care Medicine (SCCM) Consensus Conference: definitions for sepsis and organ failure and guidelines for the use of innovative therapies in sepsis. Crit Care Med 1992; 20:864–874.

American College of Surgeons. Abdominal Trauma in Advanced Trauma Life Support Manual, 6th edn. Chicago: American College of Surgeons, 1997.

American Hepato-Pancreato-Biliary Association (AHPBA)/Society of Surgical Oncology (SSO)/Society for Surgery of the Alimentary Tract (SSAT). Consensus Conference on the Multidisciplinary Treatment of Colorectal Liver Metastasis. AHPBA/SSAT, 2006.

Ashford R, Evans N. Surgical Critical Care. London: Greenwich Medical Media, 2001.

Atkin WS, Saunders BP, Association of Coloproctology for Great Britain and Ireland and British Society for Gastroenterology. Surveillance guidelines after removal of colorectal adenomatous polyps. Gut 2002; 51:V6–9.

Austin JR, el-Naggar AK, Goepfert H. Thyroid cancers. II. Medullary, anaplastic, lymphoma, sarcoma, squamous cell. Otolaryngol Clin North Am 1996; 29:611–627.

Bachoo P, Brazzelli M, Grant A. Surgery for complete rectal prolapse in adults. Cochrane Database Syst Rev 2000: CD001758.

Baker SP, O'Neill B, Haddon W, Long WB. The injury severity score: a method for describing patients with multiple injuries and evaluating emergency care. J Trauma 1974; 14:187–196.

Bang YL, Van Cutsem E, Feyereislova A et al. Trastuzumab in combination with chemotherapy versus chemotherapy alone for treatment of HER2-positive advanced gastric or gastro-oesophageal junction cancer (ToGA): a phase 3, open-label, randomised controlled trial. Lancet 2010; 376:687–697.

Barr H, Shepherd NA. The management of dysplasia. In: A Report of the Working Party of the British Society of Gastroenterology. Guidelines for the diagnosis and management of Barrett's columnar-lined oesophagus. London: BSG Guidelines in Gastroenterology 2005:34.

Bhatoe HS. Trauma to the cranial nerves. Indian Journal of Neurotrauma 2007; 4:89–100.

Bonenkamp JJ, Songun I, Hermans J, et al. Randomised comparison of morbidity after D1 and D2 dissection for gastric cancer in 996 Dutch patients. Lancet 1995; 345:745–748.

Bonenkamp JJ, Hermans J, Sasako M, et al. Extended lymph-node dissection for gastric cancer. N Engl J Med 1999; 340:908–914.

Brennan P, Ball SG, Lennard TWJ. Familial Endocrine Disease: genetics, clinical presentation and management. In: Lennard TWJ (ed). Endocrine Surgery: A Companion to Specialist Surgical Practice, 5th edn. Philadelphia: Saunders, Elsevier, 2014:98–124.

British Thyroid Association (RCPL) and Royal College of Physicians (RCP). Guidelines for the Management of Thyroid Cancer (3rd ed). London: RCPL; 2014.

Carroll BJ, Birth M, Phillips EH. Common bile duct injuries during laparoscopic cholecystectomy that result in litigation. Surg Endosc 1998; 12:310–313.

Cunningham D, Allum WH, Stenning SP, et al. Perioperative chemotherapy versus surgery alone for resectable gastroesophageal cancer. N Engl J Med 2006; 355:11.

Cuschieri A, Fayers P, Fielding J, et al. Postoperative morbidity and mortality after D1 and D2 resections for gastric cancer: preliminary results of the MRC randomised controlled surgical trial. The Surgical Cooperative Group. Lancet 1996; 347:995–999.

Cuschieri A, Weeden S, Fielding J, et al. Patient survival after D1 and D2 resections for gastric cancer: long-term results of the MRC randomized surgical trial. Surgical Co-operative Group. Br J Cancer 1999; 79:1522–1530.

D'Amico G, Pagliaro L, Bosch J. Pharmacological treatment of portal hypertension; an evidence based approach. Semin Liver Dis 1999; 19:475–505.

De Bree R, van der Waal, Leemans RC. Management of Frey's syndrome. Head and Neck 2007; 29:773–778.

Degiuli M, Sasako M, Ponti A, et al. Morbidity and mortality after D2 gastrectomy for gastric cancer: results of the Italian Gastric Cancer Study Group prospective multicenter surgical study. J Clin Oncol 1998; 16:1490–1493.

Degiuli M, Sasako M, Calgaro M, et al. Morbidity and mortality after D1 and D2 gastrectomy for cancer: interim analysis of the Italian Gastric Cancer Study Group (IGCSG) randomised surgical trial. Eur J Surg Oncol 2004; 30:303–308.

Dunlop MG. Guidance on gastrointestinal surveillance for hereditary non-polyposis colorectal cancer, familial adenomatous polyposis, juvenile polyposis, and Peutz–Jeghers syndrome. Gut 2002; 51:v21–v27.

Davies C, Godwin J, Gray R, et al. Relevance of breast cancer hormone receptors and other factors to the efficacy of adjuvant tamoxifen: patient-level metaanalysis of randomised trials. Lancet 2011; 378:771–784.

Ellis P, Barrett-Lee P, Johnson L, et al. Sequential docetaxel as adjuvant chemotherapy for early breast cancer (TACT): an open-label, phase III, randomised controlled trial. Lancet 2009; 373:1681–1692.

Ford HER, Marshall A, Bridgewater JA, et al. Docetaxel versus active symptom control for refractory oesophagogastric adenocarcinoma (COUGAR-02): an open-label, phase 3 randomised controlled trial. Lancet Oncol 2014; 15:78–86.

French Adjuvant Study Group. Benefit of a high-dose epirubicin regimen in adjuvant chemotherapy for node-positive breast cancer patients with poor prognostic factors: 5-year follow-up results of French Adjuvant Study Group 05 Randomized Trial. J Clin Oncol 2003; 19:602–611.

Gaspar LE, Nag S, Herskovic A, Mantravadi R, Speiser B. American Brachytherapy Society (ABS) consensus guidelines for brachytherapy of esophageal cancer. Clinical Research Committee, American Brachytherapy Society, Philadelphia, PA. Int J Radiat Oncol Biol Phys 1997; 38:127–132.

Gossot D, Galetta D, Pascal A, et al. Long-term results of endoscopic thoracic sympathectomy for upper limb hyperhidrosis. Ann Thorac Surg 2003; 75:1075–1079.

Güenaga KF, Matos D, Wille-Jørgensen P. Mechanical bowel preparation for elective colorectal surgery may not improve outcome for patients. Cochrane Database Syst Rev 2011:10.

Hasham S, Mattucucci P, Stanley PRW, Hart NB. Necrotising fasciitis – clinical review. BMJ 2005; 330:830.

Hay ID, Thompson GB, Grant CS, et al. Papillary thyroid carcinoma managed at the Mayo Clinic during six decades (1940–1999): temporal trends in initial therapy and long-term outcome in 2444 consecutively treated patients. World J Surg 2002; 26:879–885.

Hennis PJ, Meale PM, Grocott MP. Cardiopulmonary exercise testing for the evaluation of perioperative risk in non-cardiopulmonary surgery. Postgrad Med J 2011; 87:530–557.

Jibawi A, Cade D. Current Surgical Guidelines. Oxford: Oxford University Press, 2010:308–316.

Kasiske BL, Cangro CB, Hariharan S, et al. The evaluation of renal transplant candidates: clinical practice guidelines. Am J Transplant 2001; 1:2.

Lau H, Lo CY, Patil NG, Yuen WK. Early versus delayed-interval laparoscopic cholecystectomy for acute cholecystitis: a meta-analysis. Surg Endosc 2006; 20:82–87.

Leyden JE, Moss AC, MacMathuna P. Endoscopic pneumatic dilation versus botulinum toxin injection in the management of primary achalasia. Cochrane Database Syst Rev 2006;18:CD005046.

Lillemoe KD, Cameron JL, Hardacre JM, et al. Is prophylactic gastrojejunostomy indicated for unresectable periampullary cancer? A prospective randomized trial. Ann Surg 1999; 230:322–330.

Manner H, May A, Rabenstein T, et al. Prospective evaluation of a new high-power argon plasma coagulation system (hp-APC) in therapeutic gastrointestinal endoscopy. Scand J Gastroenterol 2007; 42: 397-405.

National Institute for Health and Clinical Excellence (NICE). Cinacalcet for the treatment of secondary hyperparathyroidism in patients with end-stage renal disease on maintenance dialysis therapy (TA117). London: NICE, 2007.

National Institute of Health and Clinical Excellence (NICE). Nutrition support in adults: oral nutrition support, enteral tube feeding and parenteral nutrition (CG32). London: NICE, 2006.

National Institute for Health and Clinical Excellence (NICE). Familial breast cancer (CG41). London: NICE, 2006.

National Institute for Health and Clinical Excellence (NICE). Antimicrobial prophylaxis against infective endocarditis (CG64). London: NICE, 2008.

National Institute for Health and Clinical Excellence (NICE). Early and locally advanced breast cancer (CG80). London: NICE, 2009: 9–10.

National Institute of Health and Clinical Excellence (NICE). Advanced breast cancer (CG81). London: NICE, 2009; 5:12.

Nelson RL, Thomas K, Morgan J, Jones A. Non surgical therapy for anal fissure. Cochrane Database Syst Rev 2012; 2:CD003431.

Ojo AO, Wolfe RA, Held PJ, et al. Delayed graft function: Risk factors and implications for renal allograft survival. Transplantation 1997; 63:968–974.

Organ Procurement Transplantation Network (OPTN). Annual Report. Richmond, VA: OPTN, 2012.

O'Riordan JA. Pheochromocytomas and anesthesia. Int Anesthesiol Clin 1997; 65: 99–127.

Park WM, Gloviczki P, Cherry KJ Jr, et al. Contemporary management of acute mesenteric ischemia: Factors associated with survival. J Vasc Surg 2002; 35:445–452.

Pimentel-Nunes P, Dinis-Ribeiro M, Ponchon T, et al. Endoscopic submucosal dissection: European Society of Gastrointestinal Endoscopy (ESGE) Guideline. Endoscopy 2015; 47:829–854.

Rigel DS, Jacobs MI. Malignant acanthosis nigricans: a review. J Dermatol Surg Oncol 1980; 6:923–927.

Rockall TA, Logan RF, Devlin HB, et al. Risk assessment after acute upper gastrointestinal haemorrhage. Gut 1996; 38:316–321.

Samson RH, Veith FJ, Janko GS, et al. A modified classification and approach to the management of infections involving peripheral arterial prosthetic grafts. J Vasc Surg 1998; 8:147–153.

Sanders G, Kingsnorth AN. Gallstones. BMJ 2007; 335:295–299.

Sathasivam S, Lecky B. Statin induced myopathy. BMJ 2008; 337:2286.

Scottish Intercollegiate Guidelines Network (SIGN). Management of patients with stroke: rehabilitation, prevention and management of complications, and discharge planning. A national clinical guideline (no. 18). Edinburgh: SIGN, 2010.

Sheen CL, Lamparelli H, Milne A, et al. Clinical features, diagnosis and outcome of acute portal vein thrombosis. QJM 2000; 93:531–534.

Shoskes DA, Cecka JM. Deleterious effects of delayed graft function in cadaveric renal transplant recipients independent of acute rejection. Transplantation 1998; 66:1697–1701.

Society of American Gastrointestinal and Endoscopic Surgeons. Guidelines for the diagnosis, treatment and use of laparoscopy for surgical conditions during pregnancy. Los Angeles: SAGES, 2011.

Straus SE, Richardson WS, Glasziou P, et al. Evidence Based Medicine: How to Practice and Teach EBM. 4th edn, London: Churchill Livingstone, 2010.

Sur RK, Donde B, Levin VC, Mannell A. Fractionated high dose rate brachytherapy in palliation of advanced esophageal cancer. Int J Radiat Oncol Biol Phys 1998; 40:47–453.

Thompson NW, Eckhauser FE, Harness JK. The anatomy of primary hyperparathyroidism. Surgery 1982; 92:814–821.

Todani T, Watanabe Y, Narusue M, et al. Congenital bile duct cysts: classification, operative procedures, and review of thirty-seven cases including cancer arising from choledochal cyst. Am J Surg 1977; 134:263–269.

van Hagen P, Hulshof MCCM, van Lanschot JJB, et al. Preoperative chemoradiotherapy for esophageal or junctional cancer. N Engl J Med. 2012; 366:2074–2084.

Verma R, Alladi R, Jackson I, et al. Day case and short stay surgery: 2. Anaesthesia, 2011; 66:417–434.

Villatoro E, Bassi C, Larvin M. Antibiotic therapy for prophylaxis against infection of pancreatic necrosis in acute pancreatitis. Cochrane database Syst Rev 2006:CD002941.

Working Party of the British Society of Gastroenterology, Association of Surgeons of Great Britain and Ireland, Association of Upper GI Surgeons of Great Britain and Ireland. UK Guidelines for the management of acute pancreatitis. Gut 2005; 54:1–9.

Young T, Tang H, Hughes R. Vena caval filters for the prevention of pulmonary embolism. Cochrane database Syst Rev2010:CD006212.